Women together
A health education training handbook for ourselves and others

Jill Bedford
Linda J. Pepper

Health Education Authority

© Health Education Authority, 1992
First published 1992

Health Education Authority
Hamilton House
Mabledon Place
London WC1H 9TX

ISBN 1 85448 346 3

Typeset by Chapterhouse, The Cloisters, Formby, Lancs. L37 3PX
Printed by Biddles Ltd., Guildford

Contents

Foreword		v
Acknowledgements		vii
Section 1	About this handbook	1
Section 2	Using this handbook	4
Section 3	Training in women's health education	18
Section 4	Working with women	36
Section 5	Approaching differences between women	52
Section 6	Learning from experience	82
Section 7	Evaluation	115
Section 8	Running sessions/training others	135
Section 9	Frameworks for women's health training	230
Section 10	Making it happen – opportunities for training	261
Section 11	General resources	293
Index		
Activities		310
General		315
Evaluation sheet		323

Foreword

The Health Education Authority (HEA) is a special health authority within the National Health Service in England, which has a remit to 'ensure that the people of England are more knowledgeable, better motivated, and more able to acquire and maintain good health'. The recent initiative to set targets to improve the nation's health is a major challenge for the National Health Service, and health promotion will feature prominently in the strategies developed to achieve these targets.

The HEA provides health education materials and other support for local programmes of health promotion. Its work focuses on seven key programmes of health education – HIV/AIDS and sexual health; Look After Your Heart; smoking; alcohol; nutrition; cancer; and family and child health education. The work of these seven programmes is planned in close collaboration with the HEA's four delivery 'settings' – primary health care; young people; workplace; and local health promotion – which carry out effective implementation and delivery of the programmes. Support to programmes and settings is provided by the Professional Development and Coordination setting.

One of the key tasks of field development, within which the settings are managed, is to offer support and training opportunities to local health promoters wishing to develop the core skills they need to carry out effective health promotion. The advantage of having trained and skilled health promoters at a local level is that they are more effective in delivering the HEA's programmes; furthermore, their skills are transferable to whatever health topic or issue may emerge at a given time.

Women's health is co-ordinated across the HEA's programmes and settings. The HEA is committed to ensuring that work is developed to meet the particular needs of women. Recognising, valuing, and supporting the wide variety of health promoters involved in women's health education at a local level is one way of fulfilling this commitment. This handbook seeks to enable these health promoters to offer health education that is accessible and responsive to the needs of as many women as possible.

There are many opportunities for health education with women in different settings. Women meet together in a variety of groups with health as a prime focus, for example: women's health groups organised by health promotion officers, health visitors, Well-Women volunteers; antenatal education classes offered by midwives, health visitors or voluntary organisations such as the National Childbirth Trust; Look After Yourself sessions offered within workplace settings or in the community; and self-help groups concerned with a particular health issue, such as the menopause.

Other settings where women meet together may not be primarily concerned with health. Such settings as women's refuges, drop-in centres, play groups, youth, community and adult education settings offer many opportunities for health education because women use the chance to talk together about issues which affect their health and their lives. Such discussions may start very informally, and groups may then seek ways of structuring what they do around health. This handbook offers models of good practice for identifying opportunities, planning, organising and facilitating health education with women in all these and many more situations.

In setting out to develop training materials for the many health promoters involved in women's health, the HEA has benefited greatly by its collaboration with the Workers Educational Association (WEA). This is a national voluntary organisation which provides adult education in many towns and villages nationwide. Women's health has developed and become established as part of a growing area of work on women's education and women's studies within the WEA. WEA branches are grouped into 20 districts, and the HEA's 'Health Education for Women Training Project' has developed work in three of these, over three years, and through this process has produced this handbook:

WEA Northwest district (District office in Manchester)
Project co-ordinator – (until September 1989) Melanie Pleaner
Project worker – Linda Pepper

WEA West Mercia district (District office in Birmingham)
Project worker – Jill Bedford

WEA Western district (District office in Bristol)
Project worker (until September 1990) – Hazel Millar
Project worker (October 1990 to March 1991) – Norma Wilson

Acknowledgements

Thanks go to:

- **Hazel Millar, project worker (WEA Western district) with the project in its first two years, who wrote the first draft with the other project workers, and who contributed comments on the second draft.**
- All the women who have worked with the project workers as tutors, trainers, or key contacts.
- The many women who participated in project training events on which this training handbook is based.
- The women we have learnt from, and whose ideas we have adapted.
- The Workers Educational Association tutor-organisers with whom we have had close contact, especially Karen Hunt, Zoe Munby, Andrea McIver, and Mavis Zutshi.
- All the women on the project local and national Advisory Groups.
- Mary Tidyman (Project Officer, Health Education Authority).
- Melanie Pleaner (WEA Northwest district).
- Workers Educational Association Interdistrict Team.
- Norma Wilson (WEA Western district) who joined the Project as a project worker for six months.
- Workers Educational Association administrative staff in the three WEA districts (Northwest; West Mercia; Western).
- Jane Jefferson (for her contribution on evaluation).
- Sarah Clarkson (for ideas, writing, and support).

- All the women whose comments on the first draft of the training handbook were invaluable in writing the second draft.
- Lynne Friedli (for identifying resources).
- Angela Martin for her cartoons.
- Our children, and those with whom we live, for supporting us and putting up with our withdrawal from their lives when we were totally preoccupied with producing this training handbook!

SECTION ONE

About this handbook

Aims of the handbook

- To be a resource for women wanting hints and ideas for working with groups of women for themselves, or for training others.
- To give guidelines and models of good practice for running women's health training events.
- To identify the skills and processes that are used in developing women's health education in a variety of settings, such as community groups and voluntary and statutory organisations.
- To acknowledge and extend women's existing skills in these areas.
- To highlight the value of a non-medical approach to health education and support and development in the local community.
- To show how ideas, activities, and frameworks associated with women's health education can be applied to other areas of adult education.

How the handbook was developed

Background to the work

As project workers, each of us have different backgrounds and life experiences and the work which was developed in three of the WEA districts (Northwest, West Mercia, and Western) is as much a reflection of this as the opportunities available to us for developing the work. Although the project has been enriched by these differences, we are white women – we have had no personal experience of racism and the effect upon women's health – so the project has had its limitations.

There is a general lack of training material on dealing with the issue of differences between women and we have tried to make a start in this area. The project has been working with Black women – specifically Afro-Caribbean and Asian women – in the WEA districts. The aims of this handbook reflect a 'bottom up' approach to training where women themselves have defined their own training needs. The resulting programmes reflect these, building on existing skills and experiences. Work has emphasised informal, active, and participative learning methods, and the events have been made as accessible as possible, and where possible has included childcare.

The training needs expressed by women include:

- having time and opportunities to learn from each other;
- networking with others involved in women's health;
- learning groupwork skills;
- looking at the practicalities of setting up events:
  - planning,
  - organising,
  - running the event,
  - evaluating it,
  - follow-up possibilities;
- gaining confidence;
- discussing 'why women's health';
- understanding health issues for women;
- exploring how to motivate women to come to a group;
- knowing where to go for information, support, and resources;
- having fun while learning;
- understanding why women-only in a social and political context;
- exploring the effects of racism on women's health;
- looking at the differences between women.

In developing this handbook, work has been undertaken with a variety of women in many different settings:

- **community-based groups** focusing on women's health, for example Well-Women Centres, women's refuges, self-help groups.

- **NHS**, a variety of health workers, for example health promotion officers, school nurses, dieticians, practice nurses, midwives, health visitors, community health workers.
- **Social services**, for example social workers, community workers, training officers.
- **Local education authority**, for example youth workers, community education tutors, adult basic education tutors, leisure development workers.
- **Higher education**, for example MSc/Diploma in Health Education students.
- **Voluntary organisations**, for example the Workers Educational Association.

Producing the handbook

In the process of producing this handbook there has been a commitment to evaluating the work on an ongoing basis with,

- the women who have participated in the training events;
- the funding organisation;
- other appropriate national organisations.

The first draft appeared in the summer of 1990. It was piloted with about 150 women who had been involved with the project, to see if it was meeting women's needs as a training resource. The draft was sent with a detailed evaluation form requesting feedback on such things as length, style, language, mix of theory, and activities. Also included was a sheet for evaluating individual activities, so that women could try them out and report back their experiences and suggestions.

Putting the handbook together has been a lengthy process but one which should produce a relevant and useful resource for many women, for many years to come. While it is not a blueprint for the 'right' way to organise training, it can be used in a creative way as a valuable tool.

SECTION TWO

Using this handbook

Who the handbook is for

- Workers and managers within statutory organisations, such as health authorities, social services, probation services, and youth and community services.
- Adult education tutors, either working with local education authorities or with other educational providers such as the Workers Educational Association.
- Women working in the community who are involved, or want to be involved, in women's health issues.
- Students on health education and adult education courses.

The handbook is useful for

- Enhancing skills in running women's health sessions using groupwork skills.
- Women familiar with groupwork methods, wanting to develop training around women's health topics and issues.
- Women already teaching women's health courses, wanting to train others to do so.
- Well-Women Centre volunteers wanting to run women's health courses and to train new volunteers.
- Women working with equal opportunities.
- Women interested in their own self-development.
- Women already working in adult education, wanting to consider other learning/teaching methods.

The handbook is a :

- Training resource *for yourself* if you are running women's health sessions.
- Resource if you are *training others* to run women's health sessions.

This *duality* is reflected throughout the handbook. Much of the information is presented as activities, which can either be read for yourself or used as a resource for training others.

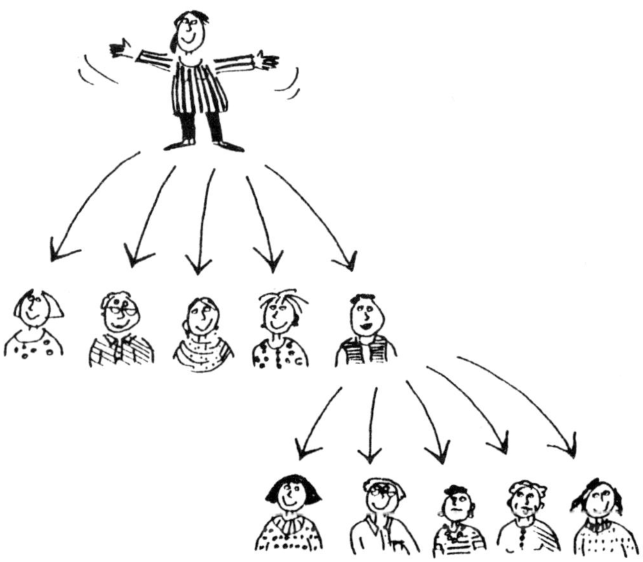

How the handbook is organised

There are 11 sections:

1. *About this handbook*
   Aims and background to the work which produced this resource.
2. *Using this handbook*
   The structure and how to use the material in the handbook are outlined. The role of the tutor is examined, and teaching and learning methods are explained. There is also a glossary of terms used.
3. *Training in women's health education*
   Issues about training, the value of, and the different ways of approaching training.

4. *Working with women*
   Positive aspects of working with all-women groups, plus some differences to be aware of when working with women.
5. *Approaching differences between women*
   Tools for looking at what these differences are and how to try to work with them in a positive way.
6. *Learning from experience*
   How people learn, building upon existing skills together with good practice for tutoring. Difficult situations that can arise within groups are explored.
7. *Evaluation*
   The how, why, what, and when of evaluation. The differences between qualitative and quantitative approaches. What to do with your evaluation.
8. *Running sessions/training others*
   Process-based activities for all types of groups, and activities to use in training women to run women's health sessions.
9. *Frameworks for women's health training*
   Putting different sorts of activities together to create programmes for different events.
10. *Making it happen – opportunities for training*
    Opportunities for and limitations of getting women's health events up and running.
11. *General resources*
    General resources and tips. A trainer's 'useful box of tricks'.

Each section has:

- contents page
- what this section contains
- how this section can be of use to you
- main content
- links with other sections
- resources

At the end of the book there are:

- index of activities
- general index
- evaluation sheet for this handbook

Cross references – there are two types:

- sections as a whole are referred to by the section number
- a specific part of a section has the page numbers included

Issues referred to more than once are:

- *publicity* in sections 6 and 10
- *groupwork* in sections 6 and 8
- *working with women* in sections 3, 4, 5 and 6
- *structuring sessions* in sections 3, 6, 8 and 9
- *evaluation* in sections 6, 7, 8 and 10

Such repetition stresses the importance of these areas and enables them to be explored in a comprehensive way. For example:

- *publicity*: in section 6 publicity is considered as an integral part of targeting, whereas in section 10 there are examples of publicity to work with.
- *evaluation*: in section 6 evaluation is considered in terms of judging success. Section 7 explores the issue of evaluation. There are activities in section 8 for participant evaluation, and section 10 includes co-worker evaluation.

Activities

Instead of just writing prose, information is presented in activity format for you to read for yourself, or for you to use as a resource for training others.

Many of the activities are *adapted* from other people's. It is often useful to use an existing activity and adapt it to suit the specific needs of a particular group. Some activities assume certain language and literacy skills; worksheets can be daunting and tutors need to be sensitive to this. Some activities can be changed to either more verbal or visual forms.

This symbol ★ denotes an activity which needs particular care and experienced facilitation. It could provoke very strong responses and emotions in some groups which could be damaging if not handled well. With experience you will have a better 'feel' of when the group is ready for this sort of activity. Alternatively, you could get support from a co-tutor in sessions where sensitive activities are being used. Using such activities can be very useful and rewarding for all, leading to enhanced learning.

Format of activities

- Aims

- Materials

- Method and timing
  - always include an explanation of the activity to the group.
  - *group size*: these are referred to as 'large' and 'small', by which is meant whole and sub-groups used in various learning methods. A large group is preferably 14 to 16, but no more than 20 women, and a small group three to five women;
  - *timings*: approximate total timing is given for each activity. With a larger group, feedback, brainstorms, and discussion will take longer. The times given are for guidance only, as an activity which takes one group 30 minutes could take another group two hours depending upon its composition. We have taken one and a half hours as a common session length. This is widespread within adult education.
- Worksheets and information sheets

These are indicated throughout the text by , which indicates that permission is given to photocopy these pages.
  - promptsheets can be written out and photocopied, or displayed on a flipchart;
  - both worksheets and information sheets can be used as they are or adapted to suit your own needs;
  - make sure someone from the small groups is noting comments and will report back, where necessary;
  - stress that women should share what feels comfortable for them, and check that they are happy about what is to be reported back to the large group.

- Possible responses or outcomes
  - all of the activities and frameworks in this handbook have been 'tried and tested' with a variety of women in different kinds of events;
  - to give an idea of what might be expected from doing a particular activity, we

give 'possible responses' and 'possible outcomes' based on our experiences;
- sometimes 'possible responses' are a summary of many kinds of events, but where they relate to a specific event we have indicated what type of event in brackets;
- 'possible outcomes' give an idea of what might occur with the group process when doing a particular activity. These have been included in order to give you confidence if you are trying out an activity for the first time.

- Discussion points and issues raised
  - are statements about issues and information that may arise from an activity. They also raise issues which may not be immediately apparent to women.

It can be useful to type up flipchart responses and distribute these to participants after an event. If this is possible, you will need to tell women this at the beginning of the event. This enables women to participate fully instead of taking notes.

Introducing training

In this handbook we consider the concept of training. We are keen to assure women that 'training' is not some rare skill possessed by a few experts, but rather that we can build on our existing skills and experiences in order to train others.

The activity 'What is training in women's health education?' (page 21) provides a summary of what training can mean in this context. It may be worth reading this now. It might be different from what you have thought, and it may be worth pausing and considering your own training needs. In sections 6 and 8 there are activities aimed at building upon women's existing skills.

Not all women will have access to the materials referred to in this handbook. If you are not part of an organisation which provides access to such resources as flipchart paper, marker pens or post-its, then it can be expensive. Likewise, not all women have books, leaflets or photocopying facilities, funding for venues, and crèches. The handbook tries to take account of these difficulties and to suggest possible ways of meeting these needs. Section 10 gives ideas for help with a co-worker, venues, publicity, general resources, crèche workers, and so on. The General resources section also contains useful ideas and tips.

Role of the tutor/facilitator

Responsibility of a tutor

There are many different views about the responsibility of a tutor within a group context. Some feel the group must take responsibility for itself and the tutor only acts as a reference point, or provides the ideas for a group to work on. Others feel that it is the role of the tutor to ensure that learning takes place, and that the aims and objectives are achieved.

While there is no one right approach, it is important that the tutor is clear with regard to the expectations and assumptions about the learning process and her own role within it. Each group is unique and therefore it becomes difficult to be prescriptive about how to be a 'good' tutor. Yet some observations about good practice can be made.

A tutor should:

- Try to create an atmosphere of tolerance, respect and equality where learning can take place.
- Clarify with a group what is acceptable behaviour within that group, so that the group can work well together. Methods for agreeing guidelines for working together, or ground rules, are in section 8. Some common ground rules include:
  - confidentiality;
  - the right not to contribute or join in activities;
  - the right to question things;

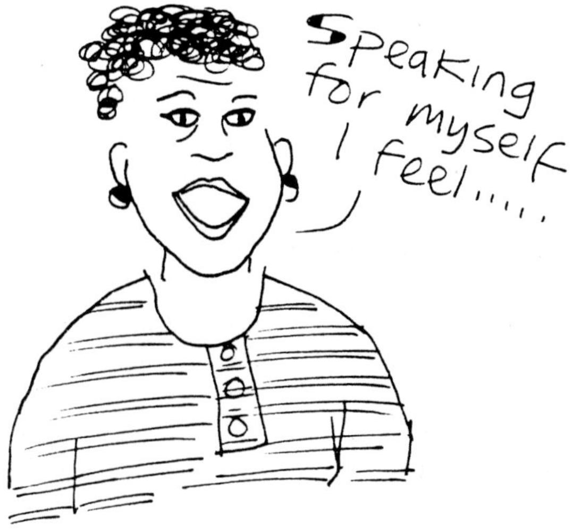

- owning feelings and opinions, for example saying 'I' not 'you';
- equal time for everyone;
- co-operation;
- not giving advice;
- owning the course, changing it if need be;
- constructive criticism;
- practical issues, such as timing of breaks and finishing on time.

● Be clear about issues and the topics to be discussed.

● Be aware of her own feelings and those of other women and be able to respond to emotions in an appropriate way.

● Be aware of women who have special needs such as mobility or hearing difficulties. Activities may need to alter to take account of these.

Responding and challenging – striking a balance

This handbook includes some activities which are particularly challenging as they attempt to look at the differences between women and what these mean in terms of women's lives. They will be challenging to most groups, as we all carry with us prejudices and assumptions about other people. Sometimes individuals, or even whole groups, will not want to examine these difficult feelings. At other times individuals will not accept that they have attitudes which are oppressive to others.

Tensions may arise between challenging participants and respecting the aims, expectations and ground rules that have been set by the group itself. There is no easy answer to this, yet a tutor will be more able and willing to challenge ideas and attitudes as a matter of course if she is at ease with her own understanding of the issues and can substantiate them if necessary. The ethos of this handbook is that discriminatory practices need to be challenged, not just tolerated or accepted passively. This entails taking a challenging role where appropriate and not endorsing personal attacks. There is material within this handbook to enable this difficult yet rewarding process to start; see sections 4 and 5.

Whilst a tutor may anticipate that some activities will be challenging, it can sometimes arise that women are reluctant to participate in an activity using a particular learning method. For example, there can be reluctance to participate in activities which include role play. Sometimes women find 'games' rather silly and not useful. As a tutor you will need to be receptive to the group's previous experience of – and comfort with – informal learning methods. If you are finding reluctance on the part of women to engage in some methods, stick with those they are happy with, and as the group members get to know each other – and you – better, it may be possible to introduce new learning methods.

Routes through the handbook

How you use this handbook will depend on:

- if you are running Women and Health courses;
- if you are training others to do so;
- your own experience, confidence, and skills.

Running Women and Health courses

- If you are an experienced tutor you may be looking for new types of activities or different ways of evaluating your work. See:
  - activities index;
  - evaluation (section 7);
  - evaluation activities (section 8).
- If you have less experience in tutoring you may find it useful to look at:
  - learning from experience (section 6);
  - process-based activities (section 8);
  - learning and teaching methods (section 2);
  - frameworks for structuring sessions (section 9).
- Whatever your current level of skill it may be useful to look at:
  - learning and teaching methods (section 2);
  - evaluation (section 7);
  - frameworks for structuring sessions (section 9);
  - working with women (section 4);
  - approaching differences between women (section 5);
  - the role of the tutor (sections 6 and 8);
  - groupwork skills (section 8).

Training others

You may need to look at:

- training for women's health education (section 3);
- working with women (section 4);
- differences between women (section 5);
- training activities (section 8);

- frameworks for training courses (section 9);
- evaluation activities (section 8) and evaluation (section 7).

Taking specific examples:

- A women-only self-help group wants to expand its aims to look at wider health issues for women. They might begin with:
  - section 4, working with women;
  - section 6, learning from experience;
  - section 8, see activities for building upon existing skills (page 178);
  - section 5, differences between women.
- a Well-Woman campaign group might look at:
  - section 9, for ideas on who to contact for funding and support;
  - section 4, working with women;
  - section 6, learning from experience.
- a health promotion officer wanting to train health visitors in groupwork skills might look at:
  - section 3, training in health education;
  - section 8, see groupwork activities (page 184);
  - section 9, frameworks for workshops;
  - section 7, evaluation;
  - section 8, see evaluation activities (page 156);
  - activities index, to find groupwork activities scattered throughout the book.

Where you start will depend on what your needs are at a particular time. However, we feel that all of the sections are essential for formulating good practice.

Learning/teaching methods

The wide variety of learning/teaching methods that can be used in women's health education are informal and participative. The first four methods described below appear in activities throughout the handbook; many activities use a combination of methods. You may come across other methods in different handbooks. (See section 11.)

The group leader will need to be aware of the group's literacy and language ability and mobility when choosing her learning/teaching methods.

- *Group discussion* is a very common method, and can be used with other methods. The skills of the facilitator are important:
  - to draw out the group;
  - to encourage discussion between members;
  - to allow time for thought, rather than rushing in to fill silences;
  - to encourage the group to look for links and connections, and to draw their own conclusions.

  If the group is large, participation by all members can be increased by splitting it into smaller groups where women may feel less daunted and more willing to contribute.
- *Pairs or small groups* can be valuable not only for discussion but also to work on a specific task, for example to fill in a questionnaire, play a game, do a role play or a practical activity. It also makes it easier to deal with sensitive or intimate issues, which could be difficult for some women in a larger group. Sometimes reporting back is not needed; in other situations it is valuable to feed back small-group discussions into the large group.
- *Round* involves asking a group of women in turn for a verbal response, which can then be written down on a flipchart for all to see.
- *Brainstorming* is putting a question or issue to the group for their immediate thoughts or ideas. It may be useful to set a time limit. Making a list of responses on the flipchart for everyone to see can be used:
  - as a basis for more detailed discussion;
  - for sorting out ideas into different categories or order of importance;
  - to establish priorities for further action;
  - to refer to throughout the session.
- *Questionnaires* can be used as a basis for group discussion, or to enable individuals to reflect on their own experiences, needs, or options. They also are useful for evaluation. Multiple-choice, true–false, or open-ended questions are some possible formats (see page 164).
- *Sentence completion* is a similar method to questionnaires, but more open-ended. It can stimulate individuals or a group to express ideas or feelings about an issue verbally or in writing, with minimal prompting or guidance (see pages 144, 166).
- *Case-studies* are a useful and non-threatening way of illustrating and bringing to life important issues. They can generate discussion on sensitive matters since they allow women to explore problems that might be close to their own, but in a more detached way. They also provide an opening for women to tell about their own situation if they want to (see pages 23, 197).

- *Guided fantasy/visualisation* is a method whereby women are taken through a prepared fantasy, read out by the group leader, or developed in the session by women in the group (see page 160). It can be a private method for individual women, or afterwards feedback can be shared with the group. Because some women in groups resist the letting-go aspect of a visualisation, it can sometimes be useful to do some simple relaxation techniques first.
- *Role play* involves acting out situations to bring issues alive, to explore attitudes, feelings and different points of view, and to develop insight. It can also be used to develop and practise skills, for example in being assertive in situations where women feel powerless. Role play can be a powerful teaching method and needs to be used carefully and sensitively when familiarity and trust have developed in the group. Some women will voice anxieties over this method, while at the same time acknowledging its benefit. In such instances, it can be useful for a more confident member of the group and the group leader to do a role play to begin with. Sometimes it is necessary to de-role afterwards, to bring women back to real life.
- *Debates* can be a useful approach to controversial issues. Whether formal or informal, they can develop confidence in critical thinking, arguing a point of view, assessing conflicting arguments, and highlighting issues such as prejudice and objectivity. Careful preparation by the group leader can make this method particularly effective.
- *Course diary/scrapbook* gives women the opportunity to express their impressions and feelings about sessions and the group. Women can take turns recording each session in the diary, pasting in worksheets or activities, or even drawings. Course diaries are also useful for evaluation.
- *Group projects* are a valuable means of encouraging self-directed learning and co-operative activity. Projects can be done during a session or between sessions. Project work can be used in various ways, for example to find out more about local services and campaigns, or about a particular health topic.
- *Newspaper/magazine articles* can trigger discussion, introduce different ideas and opinions, or provide case-studies. 'Problem pages' from women's magazines can be used in the same way.
- *Videos* can stimulate discussion, especially on particular topics. They are especially useful when there are difficulties over literacy. Unfortunately, at present there are few videos in the languages of minority ethnic women.
- *Creative work* such as collage and drawing can enhance discussion on many topics. Magazines, newspapers, felt-tips, crayons, scissors, and glue can be used in many imaginative ways, providing a means of expression other than writing or talking.

- *Photographs* can trigger discussion and group cohesion. Asking women to bring in photographs of themselves when they were younger can stimulate discussion on issues such as self-image or different life-stages. Current photographs can promote discussion on different lifestyles, cultures, and issues around the family.
- *Index cards* can have many useful applications! You can ask women to write down things on one side of the card, stressing that what they write will be anonymous (though the information will be shared with the group), place the cards in a bin, box or bag, then each woman takes out a card – replacing and taking another if they happen to pick their own – and reads out what is on the card. This method can be used for a variety of topics and issues, for example to find out expectations and fears for the event, to find out women's concerns over HIV/AIDS, to elicit what is going wrong in the group, to evaluate a session, and so on. You are more likely to find out what women really feel than if you had asked them to respond verbally in a round (see page 143).
- *Games* have the advantage of getting women moving and can be a fun and lighthearted way of dealing with sensitive topics (see page 171).

Glossary

There are a number of terms and phrases associated with training used throughout the handbook. As these may be unfamiliar to readers it was felt that a glossary would be useful.

aims and objectives an aim is a general statement about what you would like to achieve (i.e. the reason for doing something). Objectives are specific statements about the steps you will take to achieve your aim.

black often used in political sense to distinguish those groups of people who are discriminated against in Britain because their skin is not white. In practice the project has been working with Asian and Afro-Caribbean women.

'bottom up' starting from a standpoint of working with people's own ideas, values and expectations without prescriptive advice or policies.

confidentiality personal experiences shared within a group are not discussed outside of that group. This does *not* mean that group members cannot discuss the programme of the event, or issues which arise during it, but just that personal experiences remain confidential to the group.

co-tutor someone you work with to facilitate a session with agreed aims and objectives.

empower to encourage skills, confidence and knowledge in others so that they can act in their own best interests.

facilitator; group leader; tutor (often used interchangeably) a person who ensures active sharing of power within a group, who continually gives control back to the group and enables the group to tackle whatever issues arise.

good practice a code of behaviour that gives good service to yourself and to others.

'grounding' bringing heated or emotional group experiences to a calmer level.

ground rules guidelines for working together in a positive way, agreed by the group.

group dynamics the feelings and behaviour established between group members, either as individuals or as sub-groups.

group leader (*see* facilitator)

group process the stages or levels of group awareness that groups as a whole go through as relationships and identities are established.

groupwork the activity of working in groups with agreed aims, objectives and structures to achieve them.

micro-teaching preparing and carrying out a practice teaching session on others in the group, with space for constructive feedback on agreed criteria.

multi-disciplinary more than one 'discipline', for example a multidisciplinary group could include women from professions such as health, education, social work as well as women from the voluntary sector, such as Well-Woman Centres and self-help groups.

statutory organisations organisations with government funding and sometimes backed up with legislation, for example NHS, LEAs, social services.

tutor (*see* facilitator)

voluntary organisations organisations set up to provide services to supplement those provided by the state, for example WEA, charities, self-help groups.

SECTION THREE

Training in women's health education

	What this section contains	**18**
	How this section can be of use	**19**
	Issues around training	**20**
3.1	ACTIVITY: education and training in women's health	20
3.2	ACTIVITY: what is training in women's health education?	21
3.3	ACTIVITY: case-study on training	23
3.4	ACTIVITY: different ways of training	27
★ 3.5	ACTIVITY: the value of training	29
3.6	ACTIVITY: good practices in training	31
	Information sheet:	
	ways of learning – groupwork and formal teaching methods	**33**
	Links with other sections	**34**
	Resources	**34**

What this section contains

Many of the principles that underlie the philosophy of women's health also apply to the training of women's health tutors and facilitators. Training is a two-way process whereby the trainer enables the group to engage in a process of reflection and change. This shifts the emphasis away from the 'expert' who trains people in certain predefined skills, to an informal, participative process whereby participants can be actively involved in their own learning.

This section looks at:

- training in the context of women's health education;
- different possibilities for training;

- the value of training;
- good practice in training;
- the differences between education and training.

For training to be accessible to all women, differences between women have to be taken into account (see sections 4 and 5).

How this section can be of use

You may wish to:

- explore issues around training for yourself;
- use the activities to demystify the concept of training;
- construct your own activities around training issues.

The activities in this section will also give you the grounding for tackling issues around differences between women. (See sections 4 and 5.)

Issues around training

3.1 ACTIVITY: education and training in women's health

Aims

- To look at education and training in women's health.

Materials

Flipchart paper, marker pens, paper, and pens.

Method **Time: 1 hour**

1. Divide into two small groups. Group A's topic is: education as an issue; Group B's topic is: training as an issue. (The groups *do not* know each other's topics.)
2. Each group member writes down her ideas about what education/training means to her and shares with the group.
3. Each group decides what role their issue has in women's health education.
4. Share between groups. Flipchart, drawing out overlaps and differences.
5. Discuss the relationship between them.

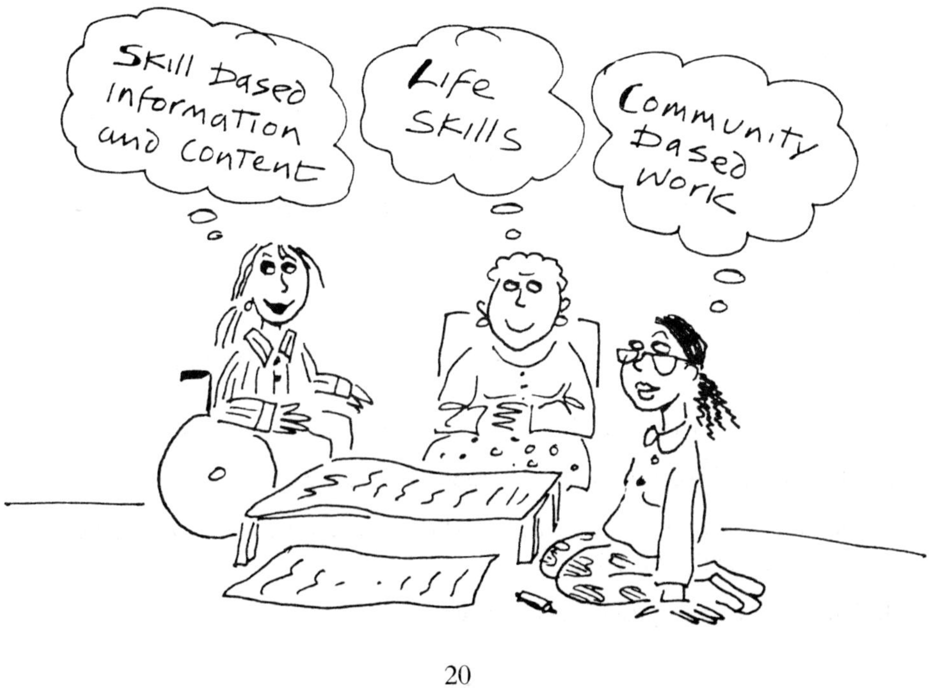

Discussion points and issues raised

- Some women view education as a broad spectrum, with training related to specific skills.
- Other women see training as a process of life-skills, with education playing only a small part.
- In health education, there is a mixture of skill-based and information/content-based materials. Discussion can bring out the labels attached to these, and how they work together to enable women to make healthy choices.
- Some women call health courses run by community-based women 'education', and groupwork-skills workshops 'training'. Community-based work is seen as for women's own health needs; groupwork-skills are to be able to work with others' needs, and are work orientated.
- Other women call them both 'training': training in the community in information and personal skills, and training in the workplace to be able to train others.

3.2 ACTIVITY: what is training in women's health education?

Aims

- To help to clarify the concept of training.
- To explore the most useful training approaches for women's health education.

Materials

Flipchart and pens.

Method **Time: 40–50 minutes**

1. Brainstorm – what does the word 'training' mean to women?
2. Flipchart positive and negative responses separately.
3. Divide into two groups and discuss which elements you consider most useful to women's health education.
4. Back in the main group, flipchart responses.

Possible responses (based on multidisciplinary event)

Positive	**Negative**
enabling	boring, frightening
learning skills	puts people through hoops
exploring new ideas	hierarchical
collective action	confusing
develops clarity	expensive
opportunity to care/share	unavailable to certain groups
stimulating, interesting	time-consuming
shows employer values you	

Elements most useful to women's health education

- Enabling women to get where they want.
- Sharing/supporting/growing/learning together.
- Personal development.
- Matching methods with aims.
- Learning experience for trainer.
- Negotiating content to meet aims, expectations, time available.
- Evaluation, integration into work setting.
- Identifying, addressing individual/group needs.
- Awareness of class, race.
- Demystification of training.

Discussion points and issues raised

- There may be negative feelings if training has been inappropriate for women's needs. While formal techniques and structures can be very beneficial, this activity suggests that informal learning is felt to be a most useful approach for women's health education.
- These informal approaches to training are rigorous in their philosophy and aims, which have grown out of community development, self-empowerment, and community education.

- Some purposes of women and health training include:
  - sharing knowledge and information
  - using groupwork skills and activities
  - getting support.
- The hallmarks of such training include:
  - accessibility (cost, language, environment, childcare)
  - participatory processes, negotiated content
  - meeting participants' needs
  - evaluating to ensure this is happening
  - promoting and building on women's experiences and skills
  - creating supportive environment
  - encouraging collective responsibility.

3.3 ACTIVITY: case-study on training

Aims

- To enable women to clarify for themselves what constitutes 'training' and what enhances the process.

Materials

A copy of case-study (page 24) for each participant, flipchart, and pens.

Method **Time: 40–50 minutes**

1. Give each woman a copy of the case-study.
2. In small groups, ask women to read through the case-study and discuss, using following prompts:
   - would this have been a useful training day for you?
   - if no, why not?
   - what might have made the day more successful?
3. Feed back to large group, and flipchart responses.

Discussion points and issues raised

- If the original flyer had included more information about the day, it would have been easier for you to decide whether this day would be useful for you.

(*continued on page 26*)

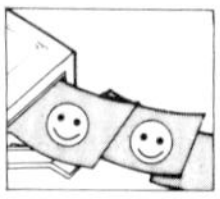

A case-study on training

You see a flyer advertising a women's health training day. Although details of the day are rather skimpy and vague, because you are interested in women's health issues you think you might learn something, so you send in the registration slip, which asks only for your name and address. In return, you receive a letter saying you have received a place, and the address of the venue for the training day.

The day before the event, you begin to feel slightly apprehensive about the day. Who else will be coming? Will the programme be useful for you? What teaching methods will be used?

On the morning of the actual day, you have problems with the childcare arrangements you have made (no crèche has been offered as part of the training day). You realise you will be late, and want to phone the venue to tell them, but the letter they sent out does not include a telephone number. You eventually manage to sort out childcare, and set off. It is difficult to find the venue, and when you do find it there is no obvious place to park. When you finally get into the building, it is hard to find the relevant room, and the caretaker cannot help.

Finally, you find the room. The day is obviously late starting, so you have not missed anything. The trainers introduce themselves, and explain the format for the day – and you are off. You are seated round a small table with three other women, and there are other similar groupings of women as well. The trainers are giving information about different women's health topics. Two of the topics chosen by the trainers you already know a lot about. One of the topics really interests you; you wonder what other women's experiences of this topic are, and you would like to talk to them about it. The information you are being given is rather difficult to take in, and you hope there are some back-up leaflets for you to look at afterwards.

After a few hours, you are desperate for the loo, but you do not feel comfortable about asking where it is. The lunch that is provided is not suitable for your dietary needs, so you nip out to try and find some food in the local area. You feel that by doing this you are missing the

(*continued*)

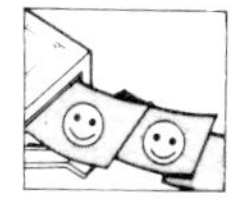

(A case-study, continued)

opportunity to talk to other women – to find out who they are and where they are from.

The afternoon is the same format as the morning – lots of information being given out by the trainers. The room is hot, and you feel restless. You wonder who the 'new' woman is who arrived after lunch. One of the women you are sitting with obviously has a lot of personal problems she wants to share, and you would like the chance to be with a different group of women. It is hard for you to participate in any discussion because it feels intimidating talking in a group of 20 women.

The trainers are running over time, and you begin to get anxious about collecting your children. The trainers appear to be rushing the last bit of the day, and in the end thank everyone for coming.

As you leave, you wonder what you have learned from the day, what the other women have thought of it, and whether it has been worth coming...

- The registration slip could have asked:
  - what you wanted from the day, so trainers could have planned the day in accordance with what women wanted;
  - your dietary needs, so appropriate food could have been available.
- It is useful to offer a crèche with all women's events.
- Participants find it useful to have an idea beforehand of:
  - who else will be coming to the event;
  - what teaching methods are going to be used.
- Sending out a detailed map of the venue – with parking details and bus information – makes it more likely that women will arrive on time.
- A telephone number of the venue is useful: if women cannot come after all, or are going to be late, they can let you know. They can also leave the telephone number with others in case they need to be contacted during the event.
- Once participants arrive at the venue, it is welcoming to find posters and arrows indicating where the event is to take place.
- Practical arrangements, e.g. for refreshments, where the loos are and so on, need to be spelled out at the start.
- If women introduce themselves at the beginning of an event, everyone will have an idea of who the others are.
- Finding out women's 'expectations' of an event at the start enables:
  - the trainers to know what women want (and to adjust their programme if necessary);
  - the participants to know what the group wants from the event;
  - evaluation at the end of the event by participants for themselves, or for the trainers.
- People learn best when:
  - there are a variety of teaching methods;
  - 'sessions' are not too long;
  - there is an opportunity to discuss and share experiences with others;
  - they are not intimidated from speaking by large numbers of people;
  - there is opportunity to decide for themselves what they have learned, and what else they need.
- Time-keeping is important. Trainers should ensure the event ends when it is supposed to, and that time has been allowed for a proper 'closing'.

- Back-up information is always useful for participants to take away and to consolidate what they have learned.

(See checklist for organising events (page 93); ideas for structuring events (page 98).)

3.4 ACTIVITY: different ways of training

Aims
- To consider different methods of meeting training needs.

Materials
Flipchart paper, pens, and paper.

Method **Time: 40–50 minutes**

1. Brainstorm – which types of training situations women have been part of.
2. In small groups, choose two of these to look at in detail. What are the advantages and disadvantages of each?
3. In the main group, discuss and flipchart responses.

Possible responses (based on multidisciplinary event)

Training situations:
- working with a more experienced person;
- co-tutoring;
- networking;
- workshops;
- staff development;
- team-building sessions;
- correspondence courses, for example Open University;
- doing the work and evaluating it;
- working as a team and helping each other;
- taking and experiencing responsibility;

- micro-teaching;
- participating in others' training events;
- day-release/part-time/full-time courses.

Discussion points and issues raised

- There are many different ways of training and being trained. Advantages and disadvantages identified will depend on the experiences of the group. Some consideration may have to be given to cost, relevance, time, contacts, management approval, and workload.
- *Formal training courses* – there are many different formal courses that are of relevance to women's health education, for example:
  - City and Guilds Certificate in Teaching Competence
  - Certificate in Adult Education
  - Certificate in Health Education
  - Open University courses
  - Diploma/MSc in Health Education
  - National Vocational Qualifications (NVQs)
  - nurse training
  - counselling skills courses
  - volunteer training.
- *Specific training events*
  - women's health topics and skills
  - topic-based training
  - skills-based training
- *Co-working* – by tutoring women's health courses or training around women's health with someone else, you can learn new ideas, methods, and ways of training from each other. This is useful as a way of training a less experienced person. (The experienced person can take the main responsibility, and the less experienced one can have specific responsibilities.) Allow time after the event to look, evaluate, and move forward.
- *Micro-teaching* – here, a group of students/trainees plan and carry out teaching sessions with each other and offer constructive feedback. This allows women to try out teaching in a safe and supportive environment.
- *Networking* – this can be a formal or informal organisation for the exchange of information and experience. A women's health network can offer mutual support,

exchange of ideas, a sharing of training materials, resources, expertise, knowledge, and opportunities for working together.

- A simple training event can meet differing training needs. For example, participants attending a training event on women and HIV might attend:
  - for information;
  - for finding new activities or methods of organisation;
  - for different ways of dealing with group situations;
  - to experience a different style of training.

(See Clarifying/strategising activities in section 8.)

★ 3.5 ACTIVITY: the value of training

Aims

- To look at how training and other experiences can increase women's confidence and skills.

Materials

For each woman, five 10-inch oval sheets of paper, four of one colour and one of another colour, and coloured pens.

Method **Time: 30–40 minutes**

1. Each woman is given five pieces of paper. The four same-coloured sheets represent important milestones in skills and confidence-building. The different-coloured sheet represents the next step to be taken.
2. Working alone, each woman writes down her responses.
3. When finished, all of the single-coloured papers are placed together, and the other sheets positioned around them to make the radius of a circle, the first being on the outer 'rim', and each additional sheet forming a 'spoke'.
4. Walk around and read them all.
5. Discussion:
   - What are the common elements?
   - What seems to be of most value to women?

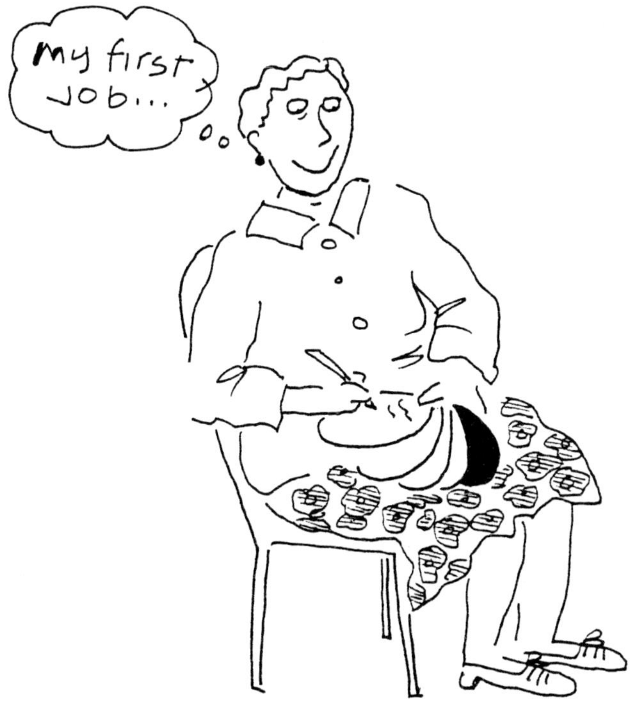

Discussion points and issues raised

- Common themes include personal experiences such as divorce or having children, and 'formal' experiences like assertiveness training and further education.
- Care should be taken not to disclose information that might later be regretted. For example, a lesbian might disclose that her sexual preference was an important milestone in personal development, but in doing so she could be made vulnerable by group members. This highlights the fact that there are good reasons for exploring differences between women, group contracts, and ground rules before going on to work on personal issues.
- Discussion can focus on the merit of personal experience *vis-à-vis* structured training and education. Does awareness perhaps stem from an interaction between the two?
- Many women feel that challenging situations have been rewarding in terms of awareness and self-development. How challenging, then, should training aim to be, given that the group's expectations may not include being challenged on certain issues, such as racism or heterosexism? (See section 5.)

3.6 ACTIVITY: good practices in training

Aims

- To examine positive and negative experiences of training.
- To build a checklist of good practice.

Materials
Pens, flipchart, and Promptsheet for each woman.

Method **Time: 30–40 minutes**

1. In small groups, go through Promptsheet.
2. Back in the main group, feedback and discuss. Flipchart responses.

Promptsheet: good practice in training

Go through these questions together, making notes of important points for feeding back to the main group.

1. What good and bad training experiences have you had?
2. Can you suggest a checklist of good practice?

Possible responses (based on multidisciplinary group)

Checklist of good practice:

- Negotiate assumptions with managers.
- Get agreements with people you are working with in writing.
- Check out participants' needs at the start.
- Negotiate practical arrangements with participants.
- Provide adequate group structure.

- Recognise that a training event is the tip of the iceberg.
- Stick with what can be achieved.
- Acknowledge differences between women.
- Do not marginalise issues of racism – gut feelings are important.
- Facilitator needs time for herself after the event.
- Recognise need for support, for example through co-working.
- Recognise own skills.
- Stop, ask questions, be honest with ourselves.

Discussion points and issues raised

- This can lead to very useful ideas about future training practice. Perhaps move the discussion towards the roles of people in the group. (See Groupwork activities in section 8.)
- Experienced tutors or trainers are likely to have different discussions and responses from women who are new, and who may need prompting, using the headings 'tutoring/facilitating', 'organisation', and 'content', to create a checklist.

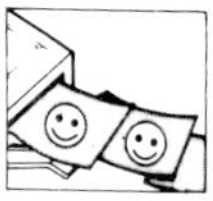

Information sheet: ways of learning – groupwork and formal teaching methods

Groupwork	Formal teaching methods
Aims usually include raising awareness, facilitating decision making, and fostering mutual support.	Aims tend to concentrate on increasing knowledge.
Members are active participants.	Members are passive.
Learning takes place through enquiry and discovery.	Learning is through remembering facts and practical skills.
Emphasises co-operation and sharing between members.	No active encouragement to share; can be competition to see who knows the most.
Encouragement of expression of new ideas.	Less emphasis on creative expression.
Group members encouraged to take responsibility for planning and content of course.	Group members have little input into planning or content of course.
Information comes from sharing the experiences of the rest of the group, as well as from tutor's handouts.	Information comes from taking notes and/or tutor's handouts.
Group members are seen as 'expert'. Tutor facilitates sharing of knowledge as well as having direct input.	Tutor seen as the 'expert'.
Learning can take place anywhere.	Learning usually takes place in specific educational centres.

Links with other sections

Section 4:	Working with women
Section 5:	Approaching differences between women
Section 6:	Learning from experience
Section 7:	Evaluation
Section 8:	Running sessions/training others
Section 10:	Making it happen – opportunities for training

Resources

see also: General resources section 11

Books and packs

Brandes, D. and Phillip, H. *The gamesters handbook* (1979). Hutchinson Education, London. £6.50.
Hundreds of games and activities which can be adapted for any kind of group.

Burridge, D., Haydon, D. and Elizabeth, S. *Getting into training: guidelines for people organising training for local voluntary groups* (1990). Local Development Unit. Available from National Council of Voluntary Organisations, 26 Bedford Square, London WC1B 3HU. £3.

Community Education Training Unit. *Training and how to enjoy it: community groups training pack* (1989). Available from Community Education Training Unit, Trinity Royd Cottage, Blackwall, Halifax HX1 2EH. Tel. 0422 357394.

Community Education Training Unit. *Assertion and how to train ourselves* (1990). Available from Community Education Training Unit, Trinity Royd Cottage, Blackwall, Halifax HX1 2EH.
An assertion training pack for community groups and voluntary organisations.

Drennan, V. *Working in a different way: a research project examining community work methods and health visiting* (1985). Available from Riverside Health Promotion Service, World's End Health Centre, 529 Kings Road, Chelsea, London SW10 0UD. Tel. 081 846 6388.
Ernst, Sheila and Goodison, Lucy. *In our own hands* (1981). Women's Press. £4.95.
Activities for women's groups and learning together.

Gawlinski, G. and Graessle, L. *Planning together – the art of effective teamwork* (1988). Bedford Square Press. Available from Bedford Square Press, 26 Bedford Square, London WC1B 3HU. £9.95
Training pack on working in a team.

Martin, Rooney. *Ice-breakers* (1988). Federation of Community Work Training Groups (FCWTG). Available from FCWTG, 356 Glossop Road, Sheffield S10 2HW. £1.
A short handbook of warm-up games and introductory exercises for use in community training.

NCVO/Information and Intelligence Unit. *Equal opportunities in voluntary organisations* (1990). Available from National Council of Voluntary Organisations, Regents Wharf, 8 All Saints Street, London N1 9RL.

NIACE. *Country learning: a development workers guide to supporting unwaged rural learners* (1989). Available from Replan, 14 Millstone Lane, Leicester LE1 5JN. Tel. 0533 517755.
Helpful guide to some of the issues facing those involved in training in rural areas.

Pattensen, L. and Burns, J. *Women, assertiveness, and health* (1990). Health Education Authority. Available from HEA, Hamilton House, Mabledon Place, London WC1H 9TX. £5.95.

Salford Women's Education Forum. *Women learning together: a course to develop skills in running women's education courses and groups* (1988). Available from Salford Women's Education Forum, Education Office, Chapel Street, Salford M3 5LT. £2.

Sheffield City Council. *Equality in practice*. Available from Pete Sacker, Sheffield City Council, Floor Two, Redvers House, Union Street, Sheffield S1 2JQ. £9.95.
Useful pack to help groups think through equal opportunities issues.

Steel, Sue. *Working in health education: a practical manual for the initial training of health education officers* (1986). Health Education Council/Leeds Polytechnic. Available from National Extension College, 18 Brooklands Avenue, Cambridge CB2 2HN.

Winter, P. *et al. Working with women in the community: a resource pack for self-help groups*. Available from Tameside College of Technology, Beaufort Road, Ashton-under-Lyne OL6 6NX.

SECTION FOUR

Working with women

	What this section contains	**36**
	How this section can be of use	**37**
	Issues around working with women	**38**
4.1	ACTIVITY: why women-only?	38
4.2	ACTIVITY: why women and health?	40
4.3	ACTIVITY: why work with groups?	43
	Differences between women	**45**
★ 4.4	ACTIVITY: stereotyping between women	45
★ 4.5	ACTIVITY: similarities and differences	47
★ 4.6	ACTIVITY: differences between us	48
	Links with other sections	**49**
	Resources	**50**

What this section contains

This section explores the idea of working with women in groups on women's health issues.

Many women recognise the benefits of a women-only setting when dealing with and sharing personal health experiences. It is important to look at what the benefits are, and why some women feel strongly about this before going on to consider training, groupwork skills, and evaluation within women-only settings.

There are four issues to this section:

- *Why women-only?* explores the differences between mixed and women-only groups.
- *Why women and health?* looks at what women's health issues are, and why they are important.

- *Why work with groups?* addresses the differences between group-based participatory learning and more traditional methods.
- *Differences between women* recognises that women are not all the same and examines the stereotyping that takes place in everyday life.

How this section can be of use

- You may want to explore the issues for yourself, or refresh yourself on the arguments.
- You may find the activities useful for women who are new to women-only settings either within a women and health course, or within a training context.
- You may be part of a women's group that wants to reaffirm why you are together.

Issues around working with women

4.1 ACTIVITY: why women-only?

Aims

- To discuss the need for women-only events.
- To draw out the positive aspects of working in women-only settings.

Materials

Worksheet (page 39) for each woman, flipchart paper, marker-pens, and pens.

Method **Time: 1 hour**

1. Give each woman a Worksheet.
2. In small groups discuss the Worksheet.
3. Back in large group, flipchart responses and discuss.

Possible responses (based on multidisciplinary group)

- sharing and trusting;
- common issues and problems;
- relating as women;
- do not want to spend time with/listening to/supporting men;
- listening to each other;
- empathy;
- time;
- fun;
- getting away from gender roles.

Discussion points and issues raised

- That we are women together may not ring true for some women, which will need to be addressed (see sections 4 and 5).

(*continued on page 40*)

A4.1

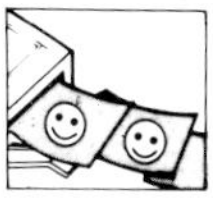

WORKSHEET: why women only?

Look through the following questions, and discuss each one. Write down your responses.

1. Does it matter to you that this is a women-only event?

2. Why did you want to come to a women-only event? What did you hope for?

3. How is this event different from one with men and women?

4. What are your four main reasons for attending women-only events?

- Some women may steer the discussion towards what *men* need to do. This should be acknowledged but as something *men* need to address.
- The importance of a women-centred setting where women's values and interests, ideas and needs are central, valid, and important.
- An opportunity to question women's traditional roles and to develop leadership skills.
- A setting where everyday experiences are treated with respect.
- An open, relaxed atmosphere where women's strengths and limitations can be explored in confidence.
- Promoting and extending women's self-confidence.

(See Activity: working with women (page 91).)

4.2 ACTIVITY: why women and health?

Aims

- To recognise the need for women's health education.
- To be clear about the benefits for women.
- To become aware of the topics and issues that can be addressed.

Materials

Worksheet (page 41) for each woman, flipchart, paper, and marker pens.

Method **Time: 45 minutes**

1. Divide into two groups and go through the Worksheet.
2. Return to the large group and flipchart responses. Discuss.

A4.2

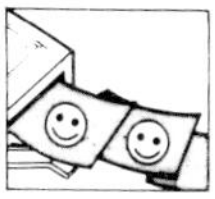

WORKSHEET: why women and health?

Look through the questions and discuss each one. Write down your responses.

1. What topics and issues are relevant to women's physical health?

2. What topics and issues are relevant to women's emotional and mental health?

3. What are the connections between the two?

Possible responses (based on work with health visitors)

Physical	**Emotional**
screening for cancer	depression
infertility	self-image
menopause	body image
cancer	self-esteem
pregnancy	overeating
HIV/AIDS	dependencies
smoking	racism
heart disease	assertiveness
old age	ageism
	pills

Discussion points and issues raised

- Some groups will generate a narrow range of topics and issues that may be problem- and situation-centred, but not include the wider context of positive health.
- The group may not see the connections between physical health, mental and emotional well-being, and socio-economic factors. Such factors affect women's health to a great extent. Class and race both affect women's access to housing, education, food, and medical services. Such factors also determine how seriously other people treat women, which in turn affects both self-esteem and what women do to look after themselves.
- Many health and welfare policies view women essentially as carers of others – mothers/wives/sisters/daughters – thus focusing, for example, on healthy mothers rather than the woman herself.
- Women talking about their health needs and learning from each other is an alternative to the model of health education where health information is presented from an 'expert' point of view.
- Women use the NHS more than men – for themselves and for their families. Women need access to relevant information to feel confident in stating what

services they require. (See Activity: how race can affect women's health (page 63) and Activity: looking at the health and healthcare of lesbians (page 69).

4.3 ACTIVITY: why work with groups?

Aims

- To recognise the benefits and drawbacks of groupwork.
- To be clearer about different ways of learning.

Materials

Flipchart and pens.

Method **Time: 30 minutes**

1. Brainstorm positive and negative feelings about groupwork based on previous experiences. Flipchart responses and discuss.
2. What makes groupwork different from traditional ways of teaching or learning? Flipchart responses and discuss.

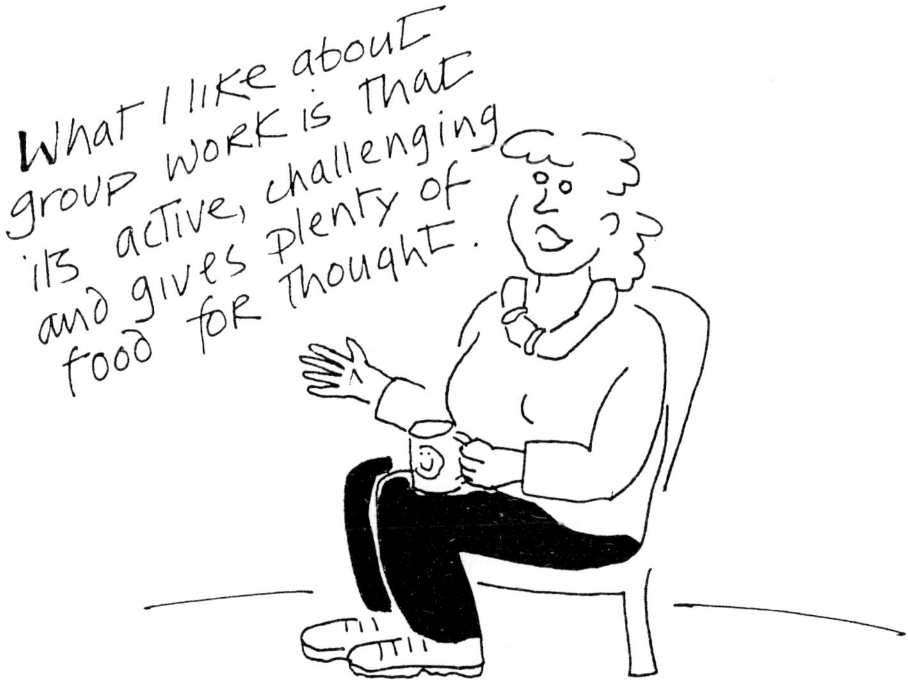
What I like about group work is that it's active, challenging and gives plenty of food for thought.

Possible responses (based on work with health visitors)

Feelings about groupwork

Positive	**Negative**
sharing	have to talk
equality	may not get answers
invigorating	may lack structure
tutor friendly	some group members dominate
flexible	games

What makes groupwork different from traditional learning

- participatory;
- group needs and expectations are known;
- actively contributing;
- doing, not listening;
- feeling good;
- others listening to me;
- using my experience.

Discussion points and issues raised

- Women who are confident about groupwork will express many positive views; women who are new to groupwork may voice reservations.
- Many ideas and issues will arise from acknowledging the different experiences of groups.
- Groupwork shifts the focus from the individual to the group, which in turn shifts the focus to recognition of common experiences and action.
- The potential for exploring issues and feelings about inequalities and differences may become apparent (see section 5).

- Women can feel part of a wider group, with common experiences, health problems, and needs. This can reduce isolation and lead to positive action.
- Learning can be fun and challenging at the same time.
- Experiences, ideas, feelings, and skills can be validated, along with sharing and caring for each other. (See Activity: learning in groups (page 84).)

Differences between women

Differences between women in a group can be seen as a *problem* because it may be harder to find points of contact and communication, and conflicts may arise. Differences can also be seen as *enriching*, because a variety of perspectives will be present as a result.

While gender will be the unifying factor, power will be distributed according to whether women are white or Black, working-class or middle-class, have disabilities or not, their sexual preference, their ages, and so on.

The aim is to establish respect and trust in a group, that is based on the recognition of differences, and the desire to go beyond structures of power and privilege.

★ 4.4 ACTIVITY: stereotyping between women

Aims

- To consider how we think about women when we first meet them.

Materials

Worksheet (page 46) for each woman and pens.

Method **Time: 45 minutes**

1. Each woman to go through the Worksheet on her own.
2. Discuss in small groups:
   - What have you learned about the process of labelling?
   - How accurate do you think your labels are?
   - How much of the woman are you able to see behind the label?

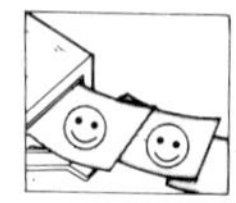

A4.4

WORKSHEET: stereotyping between women

Consider ways in which you think about women when you first meet them.

How conscious are you of:

- What colour they are?
- What age they are?
- Their educational background?
- Their accent and dialect?
- Their clothes and appearance?
- How much money they may have?
- What kind of paid and unpaid work they may do?
- What their politics are?
- What friendships and intimate relationships they may have?
- Whether they have children or not?
- Other things?

(Adapted from WEA, *Working Towards Change*, 1986.)

Discussion points and issues raised

- Responses will vary depending on differences in the group. Some, for example colour, disability, and age, will be obvious. Others, such as sexual preference, will not be.
- We may also react unconsciously when we meet someone new, for example we may expect to like them or want them to like us; feel wary of them or expect they will feel wary of us.
- How much are responses affected by factors such as race, class, ability, sexual preference, or age?

★ 4.5 ACTIVITY: similarities and differences

Aims
- To discover what unites and divides us as women.

Materials
Copy of Promptsheet for each woman and pens.

PROMPTSHEET: similarities and differences

Answer the following questions:

1. To me, being a woman means...
2. What I most like about being a woman is...
3. What I like least about being a woman is...

Method **Time: 30 minutes**

1. Each woman reads the Promptsheet on her own.
2. Discuss responses in small groups.

Discussion points and issues raised

- Responses will differ according to members' ages, colour, sexual preference, and so on.
- How many of these responses are personal, and how many are common to all women?
- What can we do about the differences between us? How can we build on them?

★ 4.6 ACTIVITY: differences between us

Aims
- To consider as many differences between women as possible.

Materials
Flipchart and markers.

Method **Time: 30 minutes**

1. Ask the group to call out differences between women.
2. Flipchart and group similar responses together.
3. Discuss responses and issues raised.

Possible responses/sample flipchart (based on health promotion officer training session)
- Age.
- Sexual preference.
- Race/culture/colour/religion.
- Class (clothes, education, accent, confidence).
- Disability.
- Marital status.
- Politics.

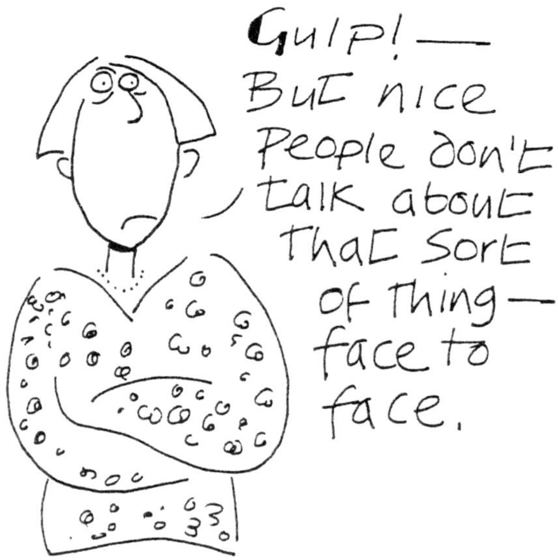
Gulp! — But nice people don't talk about that sort of thing — face to face.

- Children or not.
- Feminist or not.

Discussion points and issues raised

- Did the types of responses reflect the experiences of the women in the group?
- It may be necessary to prompt the group if obvious differences do not emerge spontaneously – and then to discuss why the group did not come up with them.
- Who has the most power among women?
- How much do we discriminate between ourselves on the basis of differences between us?

Links with other sections

Section 3: Training in women's health education

Section 5: Approaching differences between women

Section 6: Learning from experience

Section 8: Running sessions/training others

Resources

see also: General resources section 11
other resources on approaching differences between women in Resources section 5

Books

There are many books on counselling, group dynamics, and so on. Their quality and usefulness vary a great deal, but they can be helpful reading for women who have not had experience of working in groups.

Bristol Women's Studies Group. *Half the sky – an introduction to women's studies* (1979). Virago, London. £5.95.
Classic feminist book and good introduction to some of the issues and practicalities of women studying/learning about women.

Heenan, C. and Conlon, I. *Self-help: a woman's issue.* Available from Women's Counselling & Therapy Service Ltd., Oxford Place Chambers, Leeds LS1 3AX. £5.
Insight into complexities of starting and finishing self-help groups.

Krzowski, S. and Land, P. *In our experience: workshops at the women's therapy centre* (1988). Attic Press, Dublin.

Mandelstam, D. *How to get equipment for disability* (1990). Disabled Living Foundation.
A complicated but comprehensive reference book on every type of aid for people with physical disabilities. It includes legal guidelines and could be useful if your group wants to ask an authority or organisation to improve access or provide special transport.

Pfeffer, N. and Quick, A. (eds). *Promoting women's health* (1990). Kings Fund, London.
A collection of papers from a DHSS Conference in 1988 on major health issues like screening, smoking, and mental illness. Although aimed at a professional audience, sensitive editing makes these papers easy to read and they provide a useful summary of women's health issues nationally.

Pinder, Caroline. *Community start up* (1985). Available from: National Extension College, 18 Brooklands Avenue, Cambridge CB2 2HN. £4.95.
Clear examples of how different groups started up.

Szirom, Tricia and Dyson, Sue. *Greater expectations – a source book for working with girls and young women* (1986). Learning Development Aids. £9.95.

A resource book including practical activities to explore growing up as a woman – full of useful ideas which could be adapted for different topics.

Wilson, Judy. *Self-help groups: getting started – keeping going* (1986). Longman. Helpful guide to getting together, getting organised and coping with problems.

Packs

Aird, Eileen, *et al.*, Using differences to develop learning in the group. In *Working towards change: a WEA training pack for tutors in women's education* (1986). WEA, 17 Victoria Park Square, Bethnal Green, London E2 9PB. Tel. 081 983 1515.

Video

Working with groups (TACADE/HEA)
A video and handbook about how groups work, the role of individuals in groups and different styles of leadership. Video and handbook available from Concord Video and Film Council, 201 Felixstowe Road, Ipswich, Suffolk IP3 9BJ. Tel. 0473 715754. (Phone for price.)

Newsletters

Community health action and women's health network news Issue 14, (Autumn 1989). National Community Health Resource, 57 Chalton Street, London NW1 1HU.

Organisations

British Association for Counselling, 37a Sheep Street, Rugby, Warwickshire CV21 3BX. Tel. 0788 78328/9.
BAC provide lists of counsellors, information sheets on counselling, and so on. Send sae for details.

National Self-Help Support Centre. National Council of Voluntary Organisations, Regents Wharf, 8 All Saints Street, London N1 9RL.
The National Self-Help Support Centre has published a number of guidelines which are useful for new groups and women who are not used to group working, including *Difficult members*, *Leadership in a self-help group* and *Coping with conflict*. Leaflets are free with a large (A4) sae.

SECTION FIVE

Approaching differences between women

	What this section contains	**52**
	How this section can be of use	**55**
	Discrimination:	
	Gender	
★ 5.1	ACTIVITY: looking at sexism	56
	Race	
★ 5.2	ACTIVITY: looking at racism	60
★ 5.3	ACTIVITY: how race can affect women's health	63
	Sexual preference	
★ 5.4	ACTIVITY: looking at heterosexism and homophobia	66
★ 5.5	ACTIVITY: images of lesbians	68
★ 5.6	ACTIVITY: looking at the health and health care of lesbians	69
	Reinforcers	72
	Age	
★ 5.7	ACTIVITY: looking at ageism	72
★ 5.8	ACTIVITY: lifeline	74
	Disability	
★ 5.9	ACTIVITY: looking at disablism	76
	Links with other sections	**77**
	Resources	**78**

What this section contains

Women who work in women's health education come from a variety of races, cultures, religions, and abilities; they are of various ages, and have different sexual preferences. It is therefore likely they will have different priorities, needs, and ways of working as well. The challenge is to work together, while acknowledging that differences include elements of power imbalance and oppression.

Often the norm is assumed to be a white, middle-class, young, heterosexual, able-bodied woman. Women who do not fit this norm may face discrimination. This section looks at discrimination on the grounds of difference:

- *Discrimination* occurs when someone is treated unfairly because they belong to a specific group. It can occur because of class, race, religion, gender, age, sexual preference, disability, or for many other reasons. Women can face discrimination on the basis of more than one difference.
- Discrimination can be *deliberate* (overt), or *unintentional* (covert).
- Both *individuals* and *institutions* can discriminate *deliberately* or *unintentionally*.

Some definitions of the most common types of discrimination include:

- *Sexism* – discrimination on the basis of gender.
- *Racism* – discrimination on the basis of race, which is used here to denote a group of people who are denied rights, choices, and opportunities because of their skin colour. Racism can be individual (e.g. attacks on Black people; verbal abuse; a landlord refusing to let a flat to a Black person) or institutionalised (e.g. the denial of rights as a result of policies of an organisation which in practice exclude Black people.) The term Black throughout the handbook refers to people who face oppression in Britain because their skin is not white.

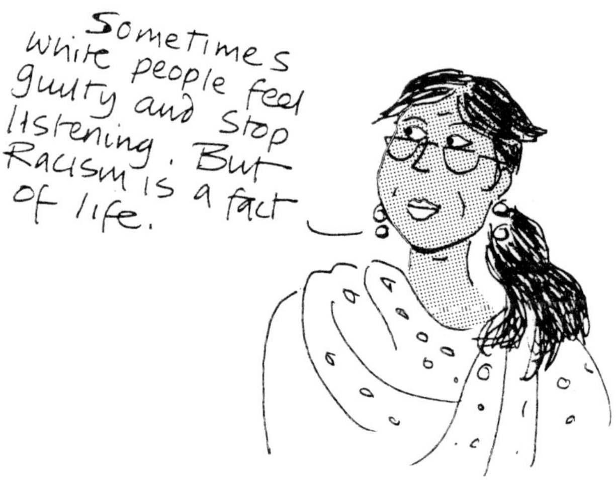
Sometimes White people feel guilty and stop listening. But Racism is a fact of life.

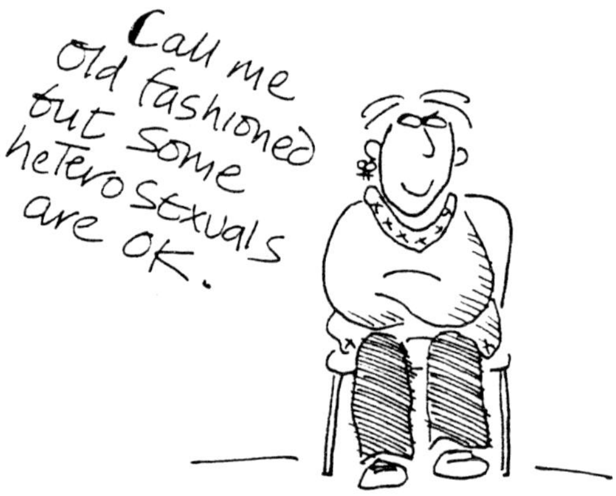

- *Heterosexism* – discrimination because of sexual preference: the automatic assumption that everyone is heterosexual; the belief that heterosexuality is better, more natural than homosexuality. *Homophobia* is the irrational fear, hatred, or intolerance of homosexuality.
- *Ageism* – discrimination because of age.
- *Disablism* – discrimination because of disability.

Women training in women's health education need to be aware of their own assumptions, attitudes, and prejudices towards women who are different from themselves.

While working with differences within a group can enrich the learning environment, difficult group dynamics may emerge, which the facilitator needs to be able to deal with positively and with confidence.

One Black woman, one lesbian, and one woman with a disability can provide a *perspective*, but not the views of all Black, lesbian, or disabled women. Their involvement in the group shouldn't be limited to their experience of race, sexuality, or ability. For example, Asian women run women's health courses, not just health courses for Asian women.

While differences based on race, age, and disability may be obvious, women's sexual preferences may not be. The assumption should not be made that all women have sexual relationships with men.

A few points about this section:

- Activities looking at differences between women can be threatening to participants, and therefore the group will need skilled facilitation.

- A facilitator needs to be aware of her own attitudes to such differences and to feel confident in tackling any possible outcomes of the activities.
- A group needs to feel safe in order to move forward. This can be helped by women knowing each other, and by agreeing the ground rules or guidelines for working together. (See guidelines for ground rules, pages 10, 145–6.)
- Working individually or in small groups may encourage women to tackle difficult areas. Knowing that issues, rather than *personal information*, will be fed back to the large group can ensure a feeling of safety.
- Possible outcomes of activities can include some women feeling they are racist, sexist, heterosexist, and so on. The facilitator may need to follow with an activity re-affirming what women are good at; action-planning activities for working on the ways they have identified in which they discriminate against others, and what to do about it. (See Clarifying/strategising activities in section 8.)

How this section can be of use

You may wish to:

- explore issues around differences between women for yourself;
- use the activities to:
  - deal with incidents or oppressive attitudes that arise within a group;
  - raise the issue of differences between women;
- use the activities as a basis of a training session;
- use this section for constructing activities yourself.

Discrimination – gender

★ 5.1 ACTIVITY: looking at sexism

Aims

- To give women the opportunity to consider their own sexism.
- To help women to deal with sexism in others.

Materials

Copy of Worksheets A (page 57) and B (page 58) for each woman.

Method **Time: 45 minutes**

1. Divide women into small groups and give out copies of Worksheet A.
2. Ask the groups to discuss the sexist remarks.
3. When finished, give each group copies of Worksheet B to compare with Worksheet A.
4. Back in the large group, discuss.

Discussion points and issues raised

- Some group members may say that women *cannot* be sexist. It may be useful to discuss how women do collude in their own subordination, and why this happens.
- Are there cultural or class differences relating to sexism?
- Would the discussion have been different if the activity had been with a group of men and women? Why?

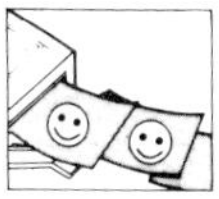

A5.1

WORKSHEET A: sexist remarks

1. 'No, I don't work. I'm only a housewife!'

2. 'My husband usually helps me get tea when we've got home from work.'

3. 'When are you going to start a family?'

4. 'She's let herself go. I'm not surprised he's gone off with another woman!'

5. 'Women with young children should stay at home until they start school.'

6. 'Women have to grow old gracefully, whereas men often improve with age.'

7. 'She won't be too reliable in that job with two underage school kids.'

8. 'Mr Davies is leaving this term. I wonder who they'll appoint as the new headmaster.'

9. 'She always speaks a lot at meetings. I don't like women who are aggressive like that.'

10. 'Women are not as physically strong as men. There are lots of jobs they cannot do.'

A5.1

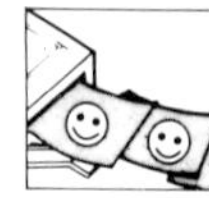

WORKSHEET B: sexist remarks with comments

1. 'No, I don't work. I'm only a housewife!'

   Working in the home is just as hard as going out to work, especially if you are looking after young children or an elderly relative. If we do not value what we do, no one else will.

2. 'My husband usually helps me get tea when we've got home from work.'

   The assumption here is that it is primarily the woman's role to get tea, even if they have both been at work all day.

3. 'When are you going to start a family?'

   The assumption here is that all women automatically have or want to have children.

4. 'She's let herself go. I'm not surprised he's gone off with another woman!'

   Is a woman's physical appearance her most important quality? Would a man be judged like this?

5. 'Women with young children should stay at home until they start school.'

   Why? What about men staying at home with young children?

(*continued*)

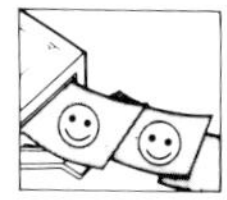

(*WORKSHEET B, continued*)

6. 'Women have to grow old gracefully, whereas men improve with age.'

   Older women do not fit society's stereotype of an 'attractive' woman. Why are older men seen as wise, reliable, or attractive? Is this fair?

7. 'She won't be too reliable in that job with two underage school kids.'

   Why not? Research shows that women are off work no more than men for illness, children, etc.

8. 'Mr Davies is leaving this term. I wonder who they'll appoint as the new headmaster.'

   The assumption is that the new person will be a man. Why?

9. 'She always speaks a lot at meetings. I don't like women who are aggressive like that.'

   If a man speaks a lot at a meeting is he considered 'aggressive'?

10. 'Women are not as physically strong as men. There are lots of jobs they cannot do.'

    Many women can be as strong as many men. They are excluded or discriminated against by male dominated organisations.

(Adapted from Tameside College of Technology, *Working with Women in the Community*.)

Discrimination – Race

★ 5.2 ACTIVITY: looking at racism

Aims

- To give women an opportunity to consider their own racism.
- To offer tools for dealing with others' racism.

Materials

Copy of Worksheets A (page 61) and B (page 62) for each woman, and pens.

Method **Time: 45 minutes**

1. Divide the women into small groups and hand out copies of Worksheet A.
2. Ask women to comment on the racist remarks.
3. When finished, hand out Worksheet B and compare comments with Worksheet A.

Discussion points and issues raised

- White women may be reluctant to consider and acknowledge their own racism, especially in a group of other women. Women may need some time to work through the Worksheet alone before discussing it with others.
- Some white women may recognise the remarks as ones they have previously found difficult to contest, and may welcome the opportunity to discuss how to challenge such remarks in future.
- In a mixed group, the white women may look to the Black women for the 'right' comments, but this is not fair.
- In a mixed group, white women may be reluctant to lead a discussion for fear of saying something that a Black woman would find racist.
- If Black women say something is racist, do white women have to accept this?
- Many women, white and Black, see white women's racism as a problem for white women themselves to take on.

WORKSHEET A: Racist remarks

1. 'Can you come and talk to our group about wearing saris and the kind of food you eat?'

2. 'Well, you'd expect Pearl to win. Black people are always good at sport.'

3. 'My children play with some coloured children in our street and they are very well behaved.'

4. 'Oh, she's so sweet and quiet, and wears a lovely sari. Asian girls are no trouble at all.'

5. 'I'm not racist but I *do* think their children hold our children back at school.'

6. 'I don't think they want to integrate with us. They keep themselves to themselves, that's the problem.'

7. 'I wasn't sure how to pronounce her name properly, so I asked her if it was all right to shorten it.'

A5.2

WORKSHEET B: racist remarks with comments

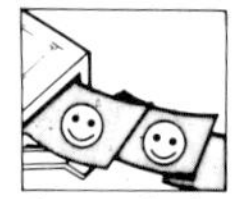

1. 'Can you come and talk to our group about wearing saris and the kind of food you eat?'
   Black women might want to talk about exactly the same things as white women. It is good to learn about different cultures, but not in a way that makes women feel defensive.
2. 'Well, you'd expect Pearl to win. Black people are always good at sport.'
   Racist comparisons are often made between Black people's academic and sporting abilities. You cannot generalise in this way.
3. 'My children play with some coloured children in our street and they are very well behaved.'
   Aren't Black children 'normal' in the same way all children are? The expectation is that Black children will be a problem.
4. 'Oh, she's so sweet and quiet, and wears a lovely sari. Asian girls are no trouble at all.'
   The attitude here is of low expectations, that the Asian girls will not achieve, and there is no need to encourage them in the same way as their white classmates.
5. 'I'm not racist but I *do* think their children hold our children back at school.'
   There is no evidence to support this racist myth, but a lot of evidence to show that racism in the education system holds Black children back.
6. 'I don't think they want to integrate with us. They keep themselves to themselves, that's the problem.'
   Black women are the *victims* of racism, not the problem. White people's belief in a superior white culture is the problem.
7. 'I wasn't sure how to pronounce her name properly, so I asked her if it was all right to shorten it.'
   You would feel devalued if someone kept getting your name wrong or kept shortening it. We value each other by learning, knowing, and using each other's correct names.

(Adapted from Tameside College of Technology, *Working with Women in the Community*.)

★ 5.3 ACTIVITY: how race can affect women's health

Aims

- To clarify how race affects women's health in Britain today.
- To look at our own racist attitudes.
- To offer ways of dealing with others' racism.

Materials

Copy of Worksheet (page 64) for each woman.

Method **Time: 1 hour**

1. Divide into small groups and hand out copies of the Worksheet.
2. Ask the women to discuss the Worksheet.
3. Large group discussion.

Discussion points and issues raised

Recent research and women's experiences provide important information for discussion. For more information on how race affects health, see Resources at end of section.

- The Black population in Britain has a higher than average rate of hypertension, diabetes, vitamin D deficiency, tuberculosis and rubella.
- Black people are more likely than white people to be labelled mentally ill. Mental health workers may be unfamiliar with important cultural factors relating to mental illness.
- There are cultural variations in beliefs about health and illness. How to stay healthy, how diseases occur, how to react to ill-health, when is it appropriate to seek treatment are all culturally determined. The logic that is based on Western medical science is only one of many health beliefs.
- Black women are more likely than white women to have hard, dirty, and badly paid jobs that affect their health.
- There is generally a lack of information on health in appropriate languages.
- Afro-Caribbean women are often seen as more 'integrated' than Asian women because the language barrier is perceived to be less. Such women, however, say

A5.3

WORKSHEET: how race can affect women's health

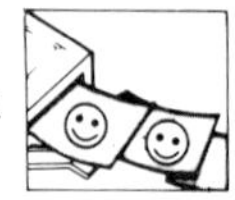

1. How is a Black woman's health experience likely to be different from a white woman's in Britain today?

2. How might it be more difficult for a Black woman to gain access to health services?

3. Why might a Black woman make less use of health services?

4. How do the health services not cater for the specific needs of Black women?

that they experience as much isolation and lack of appropriate services as Asian women.

- A Black woman's previous experience of racial discrimination is likely to influence her expectations of the health services.
- Health care workers may be unaware of symptoms of diseases that specifically affect Black populations.
- Health workers do not receive adequate multiracial training. They may be ignorant about language/cultural/religious differences. They may be unable to communicate with patients, making effective care difficult.
- There is a shortage of women doctors throughout the health services. For cultural/religious reasons it may be unacceptable for a Black woman to be seen by a male doctor.
- There is less research into diseases that affect specific Black populations.
- Economic and social position affect housing, diet, education, access to amenities, and resources. Oppression leads to stress and ill health; racism affects self-esteem and health choices.

Issues that may arise in the group through doing this activity:

- White health workers may become defensive because of criticisms about health services. It may be useful for them to consider the training they have received, and their future training needs.
- If white women had difficulty answering some of the questions, reflect back why this might be so.
- How might individuals discriminate unintentionally?
- How might institutions such as the NHS discriminate unintentionally or indirectly?
- How can Black women's health needs be recognised and provided for?

Whether individual or institutional, deliberate or unintentional, racism affects the health of Black women.

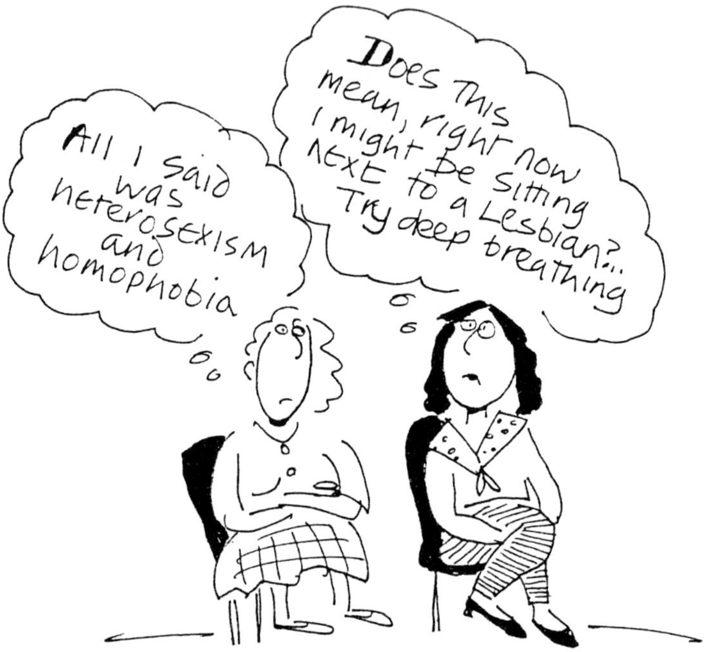
All I said was heterosexism and homophobia
Does this mean, right now I might be sitting next to a Lesbian?... Try deep breathing

Discrimination – Sexual preference

★ 5.4 ACTIVITY: looking at heterosexism and homophobia

Aims

- To give women the opportunity to consider their own heterosexism and homophobia.
- To provide tools for dealing with others' heterosexism and homophobia.

Materials

Copy of Worksheet (page 67) for each woman, flipchart, and markers.

Method **Time: 1 hour**

1. Give each woman a copy of the Worksheet.
2. In small groups discuss responses.
3. In the large group discuss the issues raised.

(*continued on page 68*)

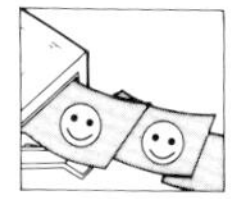

A5.4

WORKSHEET: looking at heterosexism and homophobia

What are your responses to the following?

1. Your teenage daughter tells you she is in love with her best friend.

2. Your mother tells you she is having a lesbian relationship.

3. A woman at work tells you she feels very attracted to you.

4. Your daughter's class teacher tells the Parent–Teachers Association that she, the teacher, is a lesbian.

5. Your best friend tells you she thinks she is a lesbian.

6. You notice that a documentary on lesbian mothers is on television.

7. You're in a group of friends and one of them tells a joke about lesbians.

8. Your child comes home from junior school with yet another book about Jim and Jane and their mother and father.

Discussion points and issues raised

- The facilitator:
  - needs to be comfortable with her own sexual preference;
  - should seek assurance from the group that they will respect the confidentiality of any lesbian who chooses to disclose her sexual preference;
  - should tell the group they should not assume that there are no women present who have had lesbian relationships, or who identify as lesbians.
- It is the joint responsibility of the group and the facilitator to challenge any heterosexist or homophobic remarks.
- It may be necessary to follow up with an activity showing where inaccurate beliefs and stereotyping stem from (see Activity 5.5).

(Thanks to Lesley Pattenson.)

★ 5.5 ACTIVITY: images of lesbians

Aims

- To enable women to recognise myths and stereotypes about lesbianism, and to be able to challenge these.

Materials

Flipchart markers.

Method **Time: 30 minutes**

Brainstorm – where your beliefs about lesbians come from. Are these positive or negative beliefs?

Possible responses

- The media.
- Schoolfriends.
- Jokes.
- Parents.
- Knowing a lesbian.

- Friends.
- Books and comics.

Discussion points and issues raised

- There is very little balanced, accurate information available about lesbians. This is partly because there is little acceptable research, and partly because information is not easily available in libraries and bookshops.
- Consequently, most popular beliefs come from the media. The tabloid press frequently uses the charge of lesbianism to provide intrigue and scandal.
- Other beliefs come from 'playground' jokes and folklore, and from parents' reluctance to discuss the issues.
- It is as easy to get a false impression from knowing only one lesbian as from knowing none. Like everyone, lesbians are of all races, ages, abilities, and personalities. They may also be married and/or have children. Nevertheless, knowing and liking someone who is lesbian is the most effective way of changing negative attitudes.

(Thanks to Lesley Pattenson.)

★ 5.6 ACTIVITY: looking at the health and health care of lesbians

Aims

- To raise awareness of the effects on mental and physical health of being lesbian.
- To raise awareness of appropriate health care for lesbians.

Materials

Copy of Worksheet (page 70) for each woman, flipchart, and markers.

Method **Time: 45 minutes**

1. In small groups, discuss the Worksheet.
2. In large group, discuss the issues raised.

(continued on page 71)

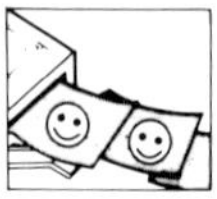

A5.6

WORKSHEET: looking at the health and health care of lesbians

1. How might not having sex with men affect health?

2. What factors of some lesbian lifestyles might affect health?

3. What positive effects might being a lesbian have on mental health?

4. What are the negative effects of heterosexism and homophobia on the mental health of lesbians?

5. How might the health care system affect the health and health care of lesbians?

Discussion points and issues raised

- There can be reduced health risks from sexually transmitted diseases, HIV, cervical cancer and from side effects of certain contraceptive methods for women who do not engage in penetrative sexual activity with men. This risk will also decrease over time.

- Isolation and difficulties in meeting other lesbians mean that many lesbians use gay pubs and clubs, and women's events. Most of these centre around alcohol, and evidence suggests a high level of consumption among lesbians. Drinking is also associated with higher levels of smoking.

- Individual and institutionalised heterosexism and homophobia can lead to stress, anxiety, depression, and poor self-image. Having incorrect assumptions made constantly can increase the pressure to 'come out', yet there can be fear of the consequences, such as loss of children, job, or housing, physical and verbal harassment and abuse, and alienation of friends, family, and colleagues.

- Making clear choices about identity and what you want to do, and putting these into practice in the face of social pressure, can enhance self-esteem and self-confidence. Meeting and becoming part of a group of lesbians can provide a good support network.

- There are many ways in which the health care system does not meet lesbians' needs:
  - Health care workers often assume that women are heterosexual, leading to inappropriate questions about sexual relations and contraception.
  - There is often no recognition of lesbian partners as next-of-kin.
  - There can be discrimination against a partner's visiting rights.

- Often lesbianism is referred to as deviant, an illness, or abnormal in textbooks and training material.

- There is little positive health promotion material on lesbian sexuality.

- Lesbians do not have equal access to artificial insemination and infertility treatment within the NHS.

- Disclosure of sexual preference to health care workers may not be treated in confidence.

- Hospitals may be unsympathetic to female partners attending the birth of a child.

Reinforcers

A useful way of bringing women's attention to heterosexist attitudes is to use names such as Chris or Sandy for women in case material. Does everyone assume the person is a man? Incidents such as this can be addressed as and when they arise.

(Thanks to Lesley Pattenson.)

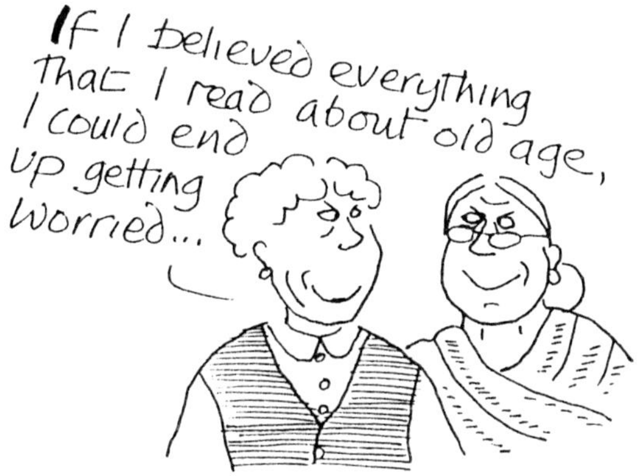
If I believed everything that I read about old age, I could end up getting worried...

Discrimination – age

★ 5.7 ACTIVITY: looking at ageism

Aims

- To give women an opportunity to consider their own ageism.
- To provide a tool to deal with others' ageism.

Materials

Copy of Worksheet (page 73) for each woman.
You may wish to give out the Worksheet as it is, or make your own using just some of the questions.

Method **Time: 30 minutes**

1. Divide women into small groups and hand out copies of Worksheet.
2. Discuss the questions that the group wishes to. Point out that the women will not be asked to report back their responses to the large group.
3. In the large group, ask if any specific issues arose.

(*continued on page 74*)

A5.7

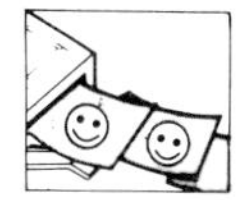

WORKSHEET: looking at ageism

1. What did you learn about the ageing process from your mother or grandmother?

2. Men go to war assuming they will not be shot. Is this similar to your reaction to your own ageing?

3. What do you feel when you see women's sagging muscles, stretch marks, fat, knobbly joints, thin hair, or facial hair, or when confronted with poor hearing or poor sight? How do you feel about these things happening to you?

4. Older women often find their needs become invisible. Young women may assume that older women will share their needs. Have you ever made this assumption?

5. 'I can't help feeling a mother is someone you have, not someone you are.' How do you feel about this statement?

6. Have you ever tried to pass for younger? Older? What privileges were you seeking? How will you try to pass in future?

7. Have you ever treated older women differently from women your own age? How much older were they? How did you treat them?

8. Do you expect to be sexually active when you are old? How do you feel about sex between an old woman and an old man? Between two old women?

9. Has ageism hurt you personally? Do you confront it in your daily life?

(Adapted from Baba Cooper, *Over the Hill: Reflections on Ageism between Women*, 1988.)

Discussion points and issues raised

- While they may have been willing to admit to discriminating on the basis of race, disability, and so on, young women may not consider themselves ageist, which may make them uncomfortable. It may be useful to look at society's attitude to, and images of, older women to understand their own prejudice.
- How does each woman deny the ageing process, for example by dyeing grey hair, using creams to keep skin 'young looking', and so on?
- What qualities do famous older women have?
- Sexuality and the older woman is not often talked about. Why not?

★ 5.8 ACTIVITY: lifeline

Aims

- To help women realise that ageing is a process.
- To discover fears and hopes for the future.

Materials

Small cards or bits of paper, pens, bin/box/carrier bag, flipchart, and markers.

Method **Time: 20 minutes**

1. Give each woman a card. Ask her to write on one side of the card: (a) her present age and her thoughts about being that age; (b) a future age and her thoughts on being that age. (Stress to the group that what they write will be anonymous, but will be shared by the group.)
2. Collect the cards in the bin/box/bag.
3. Ask each woman to take a card other than her own.
4. Ask the women to stand in line according to the first age on the card – youngest to oldest.
5. Ask each woman to read out what is on her card.
6. In the large group, discuss the issues raised.

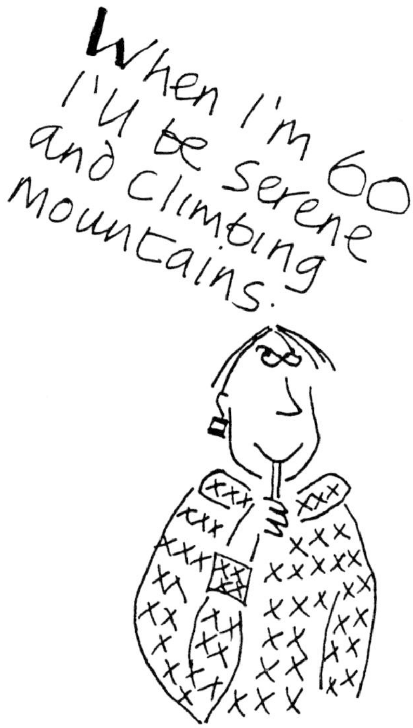

Discussion points and issues raised

- Younger women tend to project only a few years ahead; older women tend to project much further. What does this tell us about our attitudes to ageing?
- There may be fears about money, loneliness, loss, health, needing to be cared for. There may also be anticipation of freedom from family, work, responsibilities – taking care of our own needs.
- Responses will depend on the composition of the group. A negative 'lifeline' could suggest to the tutor an agenda for the group, and subsequent action-planning activities (see section 8).
- This activity benefits from its anonymity; women may feel able to be more honest when writing down their feelings than if they are asked verbally.
- This activity is useful for finding out the collective feelings of a group. It can also be used as a trust exercise, or as an icebreaker on a course when women already know each other.

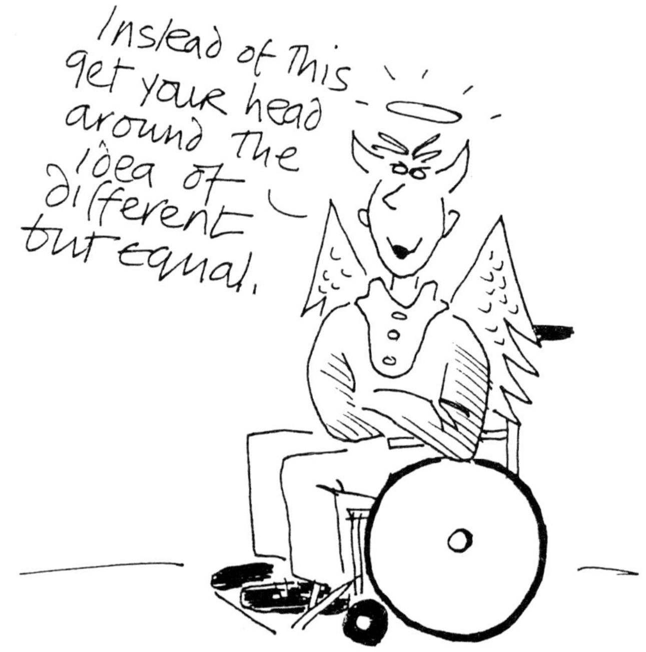
Instead of This
get your head
around the
idea of
different
but equal.

Discrimination – disability

★ 5.9 ACTIVITY: looking at disablism

Aims

- To consider what we mean by 'disability'.
- To look at how we discriminate because of disability.

Materials

Flipchart and markers.

Method **Time: 30 minutes**

This activity is particularly useful for larger groups

1. Ask women to indicate by standing up or putting a hand up if they:
   - wear glasses;
   - have hearing problems;
   - have diabetes, joint pains, arthritis, asthma, eczema;
   - suffer from premenstrual syndrome;
   - have a bad back;

- suffer from sports injuries;
- suffer from loss of memory.

2. Brainstorm all the illnesses or disabilities friends/relatives have.

3. Large group discussion.

Discussion points and issues raised

- Disability often is equated with wheelchairs. 'Disabled access' is not just whether a venue is appropriate for people in wheelchairs; accessibility for all women means catering for all forms of disability.
- Some forms of disability are obvious, others are not. Impairment of hearing, sight, and mobility need to be taken into account. For example, where the toilets are located may be crucial to some women; literacy and language may be important to others.
- What are the implications of the above for planning women's health sessions in terms of practical issues, teaching methods, and materials used?
- What is the difference between illness and disability?
- Many of us have a degree of disability. Some disabilities interfere with our lives more than others. All of us know someone with a disability.
- What is society's attitude towards people with disabilities? How are disabled women catered for in British society today?
- What is the affect of disability on socio-economic status?
- How are women's reproductive rights affected by disability?

Links with other sections

Section 3:	Training in women's health education
Section 4:	Working with women
Section 6:	Learning from experience
Section 7:	Evaluation
Section 8:	Running sessions/training others
Section 9:	Frameworks for women's health training
Section 10:	Making it happen – opportunities for training
Section 11:	General resources

Resources

Books and packs

Race

The group Training in Health and Race have published many handbooks and packs, including the ones listed here. Their publications (and an up to date publications list) are available from Training in Health and Race, National Extension College, 18 Brooklands Avenue, Cambridge CB2 2HN. Telephone: 0223 316644.

Training in Health and Race. *Trainer's handbook for multi-racial health care* (1987).

Training in Health and Race. *Food and diet in a multi-racial society* (1987).

Training in Health and Race. *Training structures in the National Health Service* (1985).

Bhalla, A. and Blakemore, K. *Elders of the minority ethnic groups* (1981). AFFOR, 1 Finch Road, Lozells, Birmingham B19 1HS.

Bryan, B., Dadzie, F. and Scafe, S. *The heart of the race: black women's lives in Britain today* (1985). Virago, London. £5.50.

Afro-Caribbean women's lives today in Britain.

Ethnic minority resource list Health Education Authority, Hamilton House, Mabledon Place, London WC1H 9TX. (Updated regularly.)

Gordon, P., Massil, R. and Rosenberg, D. *Anti-racist resources: a guide for adult and community education* (1988). Available from Runnymede Trust, 178 North Gower Street, London NW1 2NB. £5.95.

Mares, P., Henley, A. and Baxter, C. *Health care in multiracial Britain* (1985). Available from the National Extension College.
Very useful resource, including explanations of health inequalities, health needs and expectations, health services, and resources. Health Education Council/National Extension College.

Martin, R. *Being white training pack* (1988). Available from Federation of Community Work Training Groups, 356 Glossop Road, Sheffield S10 2HW. £4.
Exercises for developing anti-racist training through the development of white awareness.

Torkington, Protasia. *Black Heath: a political issue* (1991).
Catholic Association for Racial Justice and Liverpool Institute of Higher Education. £7.95 plus 15% post and packing. Available from St Vincent's Centre, Talma Road, Brixton, London SW2 1AS. Telephone: 071 274 0024.

White, Evelyn. *The black women's health book* (1990). Seal Press, Washington. £10.95. Available from radical/alternative women's bookshops.
Collection of over 30 Black American women's different accounts of their experiences – as health workers, as patients, and of health issues, for example sickle cell, child abuse, and diabetes. Written in the form of stories and poems as well as articles – this collection is thought-provoking and informative. A useful resource for discussion.

Wilson, Amrit. *Finding a voice: lives of Asian women in Britain* (1978). Virago, London.

Age

Age Concern and Pensioners' Link. *Growing old in Britain today*. CSV Advisory Service, 237 Pentonville Road, London N1 9NJ. £15.
Basic education pack for use in schools and adult education. Less suitable for women who already have knowledge/experience of this issue.

Alexander, J. *et al.* (eds). *Women and ageing: an anthology by women* (1986). Calyx Books, Corvallis, OR. £8.95. Available from radical/alternative/women's bookshops.
Excellent anthology of fiction, journals, poetry, and art.

Cooper, Baba. *Over the hill: reflections on ageism between women* (1988). Crossing Press, California. £8.50. Available from radical/alternative/women's bookshops.

Health Education Council/Age Concern. *Age well ideas pack* (1985). Available free from Age Well Campaign Unit, Age Concern, Astral House, 1268 London Road, Norbury, London SW16 4ER.
Practical pack including policy issues around health and age, and a description of 17 health initiatives involving older people, as inspiration for those wanting to set up similar projects.

Hemmings, Susan. *A wealth of experience: the lives of older women* (1985). Pandora, London. £3.95.
A celebration of the achievements of older women in their own words – looking at having lived with racism, unwanted pregnancy, contraceptive problems, cancer and political change.

Macdonald, Barbara with Rich, Cynthia. *Look me in the eye: old women, aging and ageism* (1984). Women's Press. £2.95.
Challenging book about ageing.

Shapiro, J. (ed.) *Ourselves growing older: women ageing with knowledge and power* (1989) Fontana/Collins. £9.99.
Complete health and living handbook for midlife and older women.

Sexuality

Greater London Council Gay Working Party. *Changing the world: a London charter for gay and lesbian rights.*
Excellent and practical booklet covering many different issues for lesbian women. A good basis for discussion of sexuality, and including thought-provoking and amusing cartoons. The GLC no longer exists but this booklet may be stocked by libraries or gay/lesbian organisations.

Greengross, W. and Greengross, S. *Living, loving and ageing: sexual and personal relationships in later life* (1989). Age Concern, England. £4.95.

Hepburn, Cuca, and Gutierrez, Bonnie. *Alive and well: a lesbian health guide* (1988). Crossing Press, Freedom, California. £7.95. Available from radical/alternative/women's bookshops.
A positive approach to lesbian health, including mothering, growing older, alcohol, tobacco and other dependencies. Includes a sensitive discussion of difference – around age, race, class, and disability.

Oxford City Council. *Promoting our health.* Conference Papers (1989). Lesbian Health Project, Oxford City Council, Environmental Health Department, Thomas Hull House, 1 Bonn Square, Oxford OX1 1QH.
Three sets of conference papers from national study days on lesbian and gay health issues. *Promoting our Health I* includes a discussion of the many health issues raised by local lesbians in the community.

Trenchard, L. *Being lesbian* (1989). GMP Publishers, London. £3.95.
Explores myths surrounding lesbianism, celebrates lesbian identity, looks at health issues, and the law.

Disability

Browne, Susan B., Connor, D. and Stern, N. *With the power of each breath: a disabled women's anthology* (1985). Cleis, San Francisco.

Greater London Council Women's Committee. *GLC Bulletin – women and disability* (1986).
The GLC no longer exists but this booklet may be stocked by libraries, health units or organisations concerned with disability.

Morris, J. (Ed.). *Able lives* (1989). Women's Press. £5.95.
Women's experience of paralysis.

Morris, J. *Pride against prejudice* (1991). Women's Press. £6.95.

Saxton, Marsha and Howe, Florence (eds). *With wings: an anthology of literature by women with disabilities* (1988). Virago, London. £4.95.
A collection of American women's experiences. Through personal accounts, poetry and fiction, women with disabilities describe their experiences of physical disability.

SECTION SIX

Learning from experience

	What this section contains	**83**
	How this section can be of use	**83**
	Learning from experience	
6.1	ACTIVITY: learning in groups	84
6.2	ACTIVITY: management and organisation	88
6.3	ACTIVITY: working with women	91
	Learning from others	
	Organising events:	93
	Targeting	94
	Costing and funding	95
	Where to hold the event	95
	When to hold the event	96
	Crèche provision	96
	Publicity	97
	Who will run the event?	97
	Structuring the session	98
	Final preparation	99
	Running the event:	100
6.4	ACTIVITY: the role of the tutor	101
	Checklist of good practice	**108**
	Judging success	
	What counts as success?	108
	Evaluation as self-development	109
	Information sheets:	
	How people learn	111
	The group process	112
	Links with other sections	**113**
	Resources	**113**

What this section contains

Groupwork is similar to other types of skills: the more you understand and the more you practise, the more competent you can become. Understanding is reached through thinking about our experiences and sharing them with others. It is also gained by making sense of experiences with guidance from those who have a breadth of knowledge. This section provides some of this guidance.

Included are activities and discussion about:

- Validating women's experiences of organising/managing, and being group members.
- Understanding what makes a constructive learning environment.
- Examining attitudes and feelings around working with women.

We then move on to learning from others' experiences – mistakes and successes – by looking at the organisation and running of an event, examining the role of the tutor/trainer, and providing a checklist of good practice.

Finally, we examine the issue of success for the tutor or trainer, and how evaluation can be a tool for self-development.

How this section can be of use

As with all of the handbook, this section can be read as a self-help tool, or used with groups as a training tool. This section in particular can be of use in several different ways. You may:

- want to read something to give you confidence in your own skills and experience;
- need specific information about ways of organising events;
- have worries about evaluation, and want to know more about it;
- want to compare your own organising checklists with others;
- want activities with groups about groupwork and organisation and skills in running events;
- want some ideas and concepts about how people learn.

Learning from experience

6.1 ACTIVITY: learning in groups

Aims

- To discuss past learning situations.
- To help women to become aware of group and learning processes.
- To validate women's experiences and promote confidence.

Materials

Worksheet (page 85) for each woman, flipchart, paper, and pens.

Method **Time: 2 hours**

1. In large group brainstorm what groups women have belonged to. Flipchart responses.
2. In small groups, go through Worksheet.
3. In the large group, report back, flipchart and discuss.

Possible responses (based on working with health visitor students)

Brainstorm:

groups women belong to:

- family groups;
- social groups;
- work teams;
- campaigning groups;
- therapy groups;
- student groups;
- mother and toddler groups;
- political groups;
- down the pub.

(*continued on page 86*)

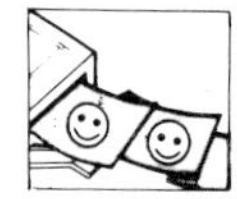

A6.1

WORKSHEET: learning in groups

1. There is a huge range of learning situations, from informal discussion through to formal lecturing. What types have you experienced?

2. In which situations have learning and self-development been most helped? What has made it hard to learn?

3. Have you ever had to help someone to learn or to develop a skill? How did you approach it?

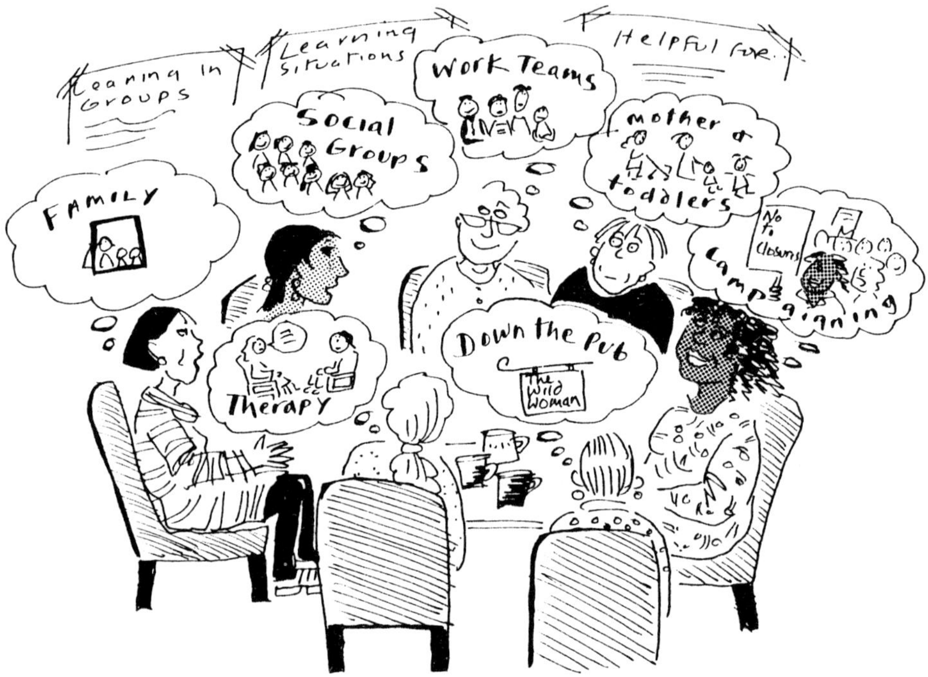

Learning situations:

- peer groups;
- reading;
- TV;
- talking and discussing;
- formal education institutions;
- support groups;
- supervision;
- experimenting for self;
- adult education.

Helpful for learning:

- feeling involved, supported;
- relevant information;

- no waffle;
- able to say 'Haven't a clue';
- okay to make mistakes;
- able to go at own pace;
- good communication;
- participatory;
- feeling warm enough and comfortable.

Unhelpful for learning:
- noisy;
- too formal, too many people in group;
- trying to write and listen at the same time;
- unable to ask questions;
- assessed in rigid way;
- too much waffle and padding;
- tutor not knowing subject.

Passing on skills:
- find out what person already knows;
- show/give person information and let them get on with it;
- be clear;
- check out that person understands;
- let them try to do it – do not do it for them;
- retreat to safe distance – but be there if they ask for help;
- be prepared for them to do it differently.

Discussion points and issues raised

- Women who have not examined these issues before will want to talk longer than those who have.

- You do not have to be a group leader to have valuable experiences in groupwork. You do not have to be a tutor to understand how people learn – you can do it by being a participant. However, some information and understanding of theories do help. For example, there is a theory that people learn and remember more if they have played an active part in the learning process. (See the information sheet 'How people learn' page 111.)
- Experience does not always equal understanding: reading or learning about the theory of groupwork and learning methods can promote understanding and make sense of personal experiences. For example, theory about the stages groups go through can illuminate group experiences and help explain the way a certain group acted. (See the information sheet 'The group process', page 112.)
- Experiences gained in one setting can be transferred to others, such as a women's health tutor training others to tutor women's health (see section 8).
- While some people prefer a lecture-type delivery of information, a formal approach does not always equal professionalism or competence.
- Informal, relaxed, and comfortable settings, together with clear aims, good structure, and appropriate facilitation can promote greater participation and produce greater depth of learning.
- Any situation can block learning, such as chairs in formal rows; distracting noises; uncertainty; having to perform.
- The passing on of skills happens every day, and to some extent we all have this ability. Whilst there are specific groupwork skills that need to be learnt, we all have some idea about what makes good and bad learning situations and this needs to be built upon. A handbook like this can do only so much towards this. There are a variety of courses available which can provide supportive structures for taking these ideas a step further; for example, health education certificate/diploma/MSc courses; various Open University courses about health and groupwork, and so on. (See section 3 and groupwork activities in section 8.)

6.2 ACTIVITY: management and organisation

Aims

- To validate women's life experiences.
- To acknowledge how women manage and organise every day.
- To promote this and use it for women's self-development.

Materials

Flipchart, pens, and Worksheet (page 90) for each woman.

Method **Time: 1 hour**

1. In small groups, read and discuss the Worksheet.
2. In the large group, report back main points (not details). Flipchart responses.
3. Discuss.

Possible responses

Main points of interest:

- Never thought of myself as superwoman before!
- Tires me out just to think about it.
- Do it automatically.
- Things need to change!
- I must be an expert juggler by now!
- How do we change it?

Discussion points and issues raised

- Management and organisation take up a large part of women's everyday lives. They bond women together and show some of the similarities between women in different situations.
- Management can mean doing the best you can with the resources you have, such as:
  - materials (including money);
  - equipment;
  - people and support;
  - time;
  - skills and training;
  - aims and objectives.
- Priorities, choices, and delegation are important in managing and organising. If you identified many strands in your life, by looking at business management you could review your commitments, aims, and expectations, and start to prioritise to make changes.

(*continued on page 91*)

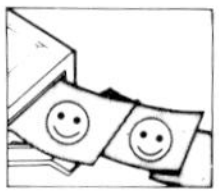

A6.2

WORKSHEET: management and organisation

1. Do you live with other people/children and look after some of their needs?

2. Do you co-ordinate daily activities such as:
   - arranging transport;
   - organising work rotas;
   - getting children off to school;
   - other things.

3. Does your work involve organising yourself?

4. Do you supervise or manage others?

5. Do you juggle with all of this, managing several strands in your life? What are they?

- What information and support would you need to do this?
- Tutoring and training involve foreseeing and clarifying people's needs, having clear aims and objectives, and preparing and carrying out activities in an appropriate way.

(See activities for building on existing skills in section 8.)

6.3 ACTIVITY: working with women

Aims
- To understand the value of women-only settings for health education.

Materials
Flipchart, pens, and Worksheet (page 92) for each woman.

Method **Time: 1 hour**

1. In the large group brainstorm: what associations or connections do you have or have you had to other women.
2. In small groups, go through the Worksheet.
3. Report back, discuss in large group, flipchart.

Possible responses

Brainstorm:
- all girls' school;
- sisters;
- play lots of sport with women;
- Well-Women worker;
- health visitor;
- rape crisis worker;
- run a playgroup, meet mums;
- midwife;
- member of a women's group;

(*continued on page 93*)

A6.3

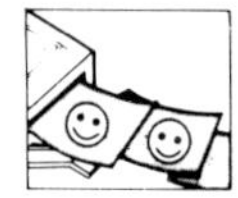

WORKSHEET: working with women

1. How important are your connections with other women?

2. What do you think women talk about in all-women groups? How does this relate to health education?

3. When women are working together, how important are the differences that exist between them?

4. How do these differences affect self-esteem or self-confidence?

- work with women;
- women friends.

Discussion points and issues raised

- It can be useful to see what our attitudes are to women before starting to work in women-only settings.
- Some women will have many more connections with women than others, which will reflect different lifestyles and choices.
- Women will have both negative and positive experiences of working within all-women groups. What were the different situations, and what led to these feelings?
- The potential of women-only groups may not be realised because of differences, lack of confidentiality, jealousy and many other factors. Women's groups have the same problems as other groups, but the potential to work through these is different from other groups.
- Some women may have tried to work with women and now feel it is not worth it.
  - What were they trying to do? How did they go about it?
  - Was it what women wanted or what others thought would be good for them?

(See sections 4 and 6.)

Learning from others

Organising events

Have you ever been involved in events where things have gone wrong, like:

- the date or time on the leaflet was incorrect;
- the car park was being resurfaced and there was nowhere else to park;
- it was an in-service teacher training day and loads more children turned up;
- all the children were under one-year-old;
- the toilets were not working;
- all the windows were jammed and it was really hot and sunny;

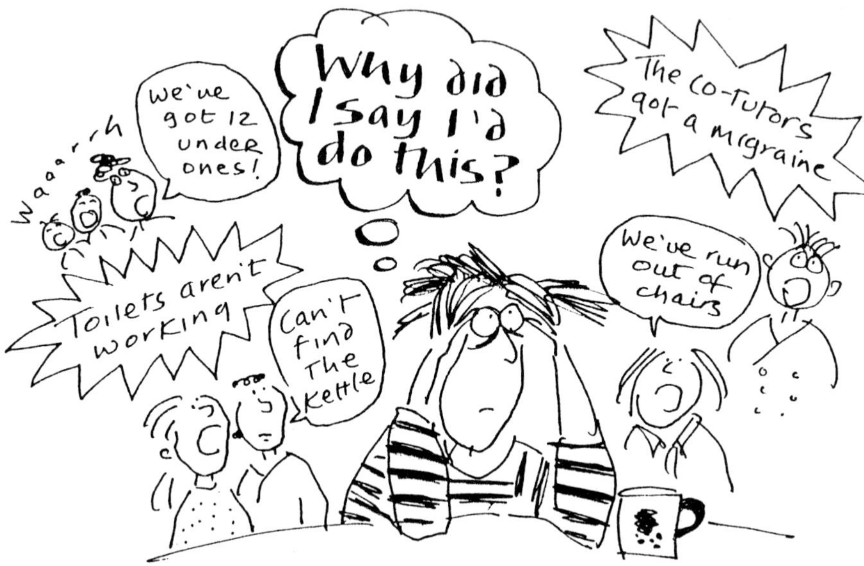
Why did I say I'd do this?
We've got 12 under ones!
Waaaarrh
The co-tutors got a migraine
Toilets aren't working
Can't find the kettle
We've run out of chairs

- people were peering through the glass doors;
- the cups and kettle were locked away;
- there were not enough chairs (or the room was half-full of stacked chairs);
- the co-tutor was two hours late.

All of the above are related to preparation and organisation, which is what this part of the section looks at in detail. It includes a lot of checklists. Try going through them and asking yourself:

- Is this relevant to what I want to do?
- Do I do this already? If not, why not?

Checklists are never complete. You will probably want to add to them as your experience of groupwork grows.

Targeting
The first thing to think about is *who is the event for.* This is called targeting, and will determine your planning and preparation. Different women have different needs, interests, experiences and opportunities, and will respond to such things as publicity and choice of venue in equally different ways.

Targeting will affect the preparation and organisation of:

- costing and funding
- where and when to hold the event
- the need for a crèche
- what type of publicity to use
- who will run the event
- what type of activities to use and what to avoid

Costing and funding

Your costs may include: room hire, heating, publicity, paying tutor/facilitator, photocopying, resources, childcare.

How will these costs be met? Will other organisations and agencies meet some of the costs or will participants pay them all?

Will they be able to pay, or will this stop them from coming?

To encourage women to come, should the event then be free? (See section 10.)

Where to hold the event

When deciding on the venue, think about the following:

- Is it acceptable to the target group? For example, a GP's surgery is not appropriate for women who rarely see, or have had bad experiences of, their GP.
- Whether it is near bus routes or train stations will affect the target groups. Does it rely on having a car or spending a lot on fares?
- Has it got wheelchair access?
- Is it well-lit and near busy places? Evening sessions can be scary and dangerous for women.
- Is it comfortable and warm? See the venue beforehand and make contact with the caretaker to foster a good relationship.
- Check toilets, room size, and kitchen facilities.
- Has it got a crèche room with crèche workers; can you use the equipment?
- Do you need to book any equipment in advance?
- Is it free or do you have to pay? Can you negotiate?
- Always confirm bookings in writing, stating your exact needs, and keep a copy.

When to hold the event

- Weekday or weekend? Women in paid work with supportive managers prefer weekday events within their normal working time. However, if they find it hard to get paid time for training, they may choose to attend weekend events. Unwaged women may prefer weekday events while their children are at school, but weekends may be easier if their partners can provide childcare. Part-time workers usually have to attend training in their own time.
- Should it be Saturday or Sunday? Different cultures and peer groups use weekends in different ways. Different religions and cultures recognise festivals throughout the years. (See calendar of religious festival, section 10, page 289.)
- Daytime or evening? Think about the target group: do you want women in paid daytime work, women working twilight shifts, or women doing unpaid work at home?
- For women with children, weekday daytime sessions have to end before school or nursery finishes.
- Check school times, in-service training for teachers, local holidays.
- If it is during work time and is a work-based event, then liaise with management to set up cover for participants. (This can take ages!)
- Women may need to re-schedule workloads or clear with line managers to arrange for paying for training. Allow about two months for this.

Crèche provision

- Has the venue got a crèche you can use? What is the capacity and cost, and does the timing fit in with the session?
- Is there a room a crèche can use? You should check with local Social Services for updated health and safety regulations.
- What equipment and materials will you need? Check with crèche workers about this.
- Find out the crèche needs of the participants. (See pages 283–4 for sample crèche form.)
- Inform crèche workers of numbers and details of children at least a week in advance.

- Check legal requirements of ratios of adults to children through your local Social Services Department. As a guideline these are:

12 weeks to 1 year old	1 adult to 3 children
1 to 2 years old	1 adult to 3 children
2 to 3 years old	1 adult to 4 children
3 to 5 years old	1 adult to 5 children
over 5 years old	1 adult to 8 children

For good practice there should always be at least two crèche workers to enable visits to the loo, and so on.

Publicity

- What type of publicity is most appropriate to your target group? Leaflets, posters, face-to-face, radio, personal letters, word-of-mouth? What about a mixture?
- Pre-registration. A tear-off slip to return with name, address, and phone number, interest in attending and crèche needs. Do not forget to give a return address!
- What kind of language and style? Wordy or cartoons? What level of English or literacy are you assuming for your target group?

(See Publicity, section 10.)

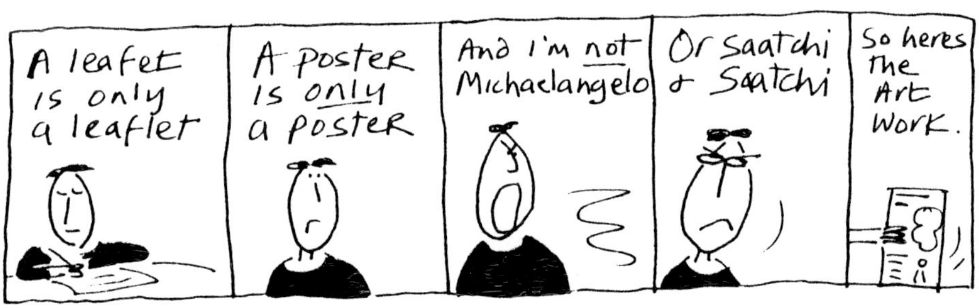
A leafet is only a leaflet
A poster is only a poster
And I'm not Michaelangelo
Or Saatchi & Saatchi
So heres the Art Work.

Who will run the event?

- If you are co-tutoring, organise time to meet or share aims, assumptions, and to plan the event. Also plan for time after the event to evaluate both the event and each other's contributions. (See sections 8 and 10.)

- What support, extra training, or other resources do you or your co-tutor need? Be aware of your own skills, experiences, and limitations.
- Be clear about what type of person is best suited to work with a particular group. The tutor has to be acceptable to, and credible with the participants.

Structuring the session

- Some common elements to a session include:
  - introductions, expectations, ground rules;
  - setting agendas and negotiating content;
  - tea/coffee breaks;
  - enliveners and mood-changers;
  - review of session;
  - evaluation;
  - taking things forward/follow-up;
  - bringing group to a balanced close.
- Negotiating and finding out what women want in the session can be done via pre-registration forms or at the start of the event.
- How long is the session/event?
  - How much time is needed for introductions, expectations and evaluation?
  - How much for adequate breaks for tea and lunch?
- Is it a one-off or the start of a course?
  - Time given to negotiating content will vary.
  - Is there a need to impose/shortcut ground rules, or, given time limitations, can they be obtained from the group?
- What is the session about?
  - Aims of the session will affect the learning methods used.
  - What is the balance between activities and information-giving?
  - Whether or not sessions are fact-based and noncontroversial, ground rules are necessary because the process of groupwork means that you never know beforehand the depth of feelings that might surface.

  (See groupwork activities in section 8; and section 9.)
- Which learning methods? Are they appropriate to the group, topic, and length of session?

  (See section 2.)

Final preparation

- Venue
  - check the booking
  - provide the signs showing where to go
  - arrange seating (maybe in a circle rather than rows)
  - check any equipment booked is available
  - check refreshments and access to loos and kitchen.
- Organise resources such as books, leaflets, flipcharts.
- Check tutor or co-tutor can come at the appointed time.
- Check room and equipment for crèche, and crèche workers okay.
- Have back-up activities to use in case you get through everything in record time.
- Checklist of what to take:
  - flipchart paper and pens
  - spare paper pads
  - Blu-tack
  - name labels
  - scissors
  - Post-its
  - spare pens
  - own notes
  - resources
  - handouts
  - evaluation sheets and SAEs, if needed
  - refreshments and nibbles, if needed

Check what others have done:

- It is vital that you have confidence in the people you are working with and who you are dependent upon for some aspects of planning.
- If you are initiating the event, be clear about what is arranged with others – room bookings and so on.
- If you are tutoring or training on events that others have set up, ask the questions you need. Check what has already been organised and clear up such things as timing for breaks, childcare provision, and so on.

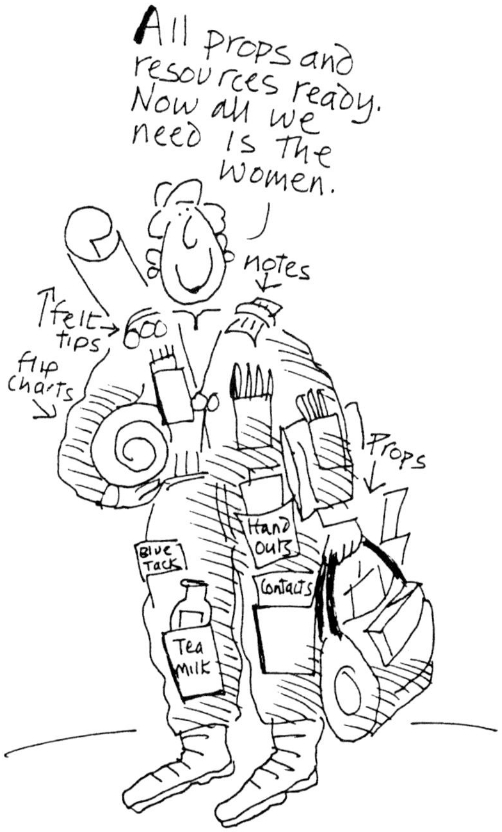

Running the event

It is worth accepting before the event that no matter how well you plan, there is always the possibility of something not going according to plan.

For example:

- Women leave before the end of the session.
- One woman or a small clique take over the discussion and the rest of the group shuts up.
- One woman shares very personal experiences and everyone responds with embarrassed silence.
- Previous antagonisms arise within the group. (This might occur within small communities and rural areas.)

- Other hidden agendas within the group that you know nothing about.

How you cope with such things depends on how you see the tutor's role in relation to the group.

6.4 ACTIVITY: the role of the tutor

Aims
- To examine the tutor's/trainer's role.
- To identify ways of dealing with difficult situations in groups.

Materials
Flipchart, pens, and Worksheet (page 102) for each woman.

Method **Time: 1½ hours**

1. Brainstorm difficult situations in groups, either as tutor or participant.
2. Work in small groups, with two case studies (see pages 102–3) per group.
3. Report back and discuss in large group.

Possible responses (based on multidisciplinary group)
Brainstorm:
- talkative women and quiet women;
- latecomers and early leavers;
- lack of group response;
- emotions erupting;
- differences between women;
- insensitivity;
- expectations not being met;
- uncertainty about how much to disclose;
- sharing and then feeling vulnerable;
- resistance to participatory learning;
- wanting tutor to be expert.

(*continued on page 104*)

A6.4

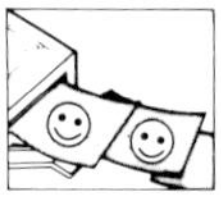

WORKSHEET: case-studies of the role of the tutor

1. A woman in the group tells you she has a lump in her breast. She seems to want reassurance that it is not cancer.
   - How will you respond?
   - Is it fair to expect medical knowledge from a tutor?

2. During a session, a woman says she feels so depressed she is thinking of killing herself.
   - How do you feel?
   - Can you help her? How much?
   - What counselling skills do you have?

3. After a session, a woman asks you for the number of a women's refuge because her husband is battering her. You give her the number. The following week she stays behind and asks you to help her to get an injunction against her husband.
   - What can you do?
   - Do you have the knowledge to get involved?
   - Are tutors social workers or Women's Aid workers?

4. It is the first session of a new course and the group wants information, not discussion. They see you as the expert, giving them the facts.
   - How would you deal with this situation?

(*continued*)

(*Worksheet, continued*)

5. Three talkative women dominate the group. Frequently the session either runs over or you have to leave bits out, and it always ends on a rushed note.
   - How might you keep the talkative women to the time limit?
   - What about the quieter women who let them talk? What can be done for them?

6. You are running a session on menopause and one woman bursts into tears and tells the group about her own struggles with this. Everyone sits in silence and embarrassment at such strength of emotion.
   - What would you feel like?
   - What is the best thing to do?
   - Is there a difference between a training group within a work setting and a community-based women's health group?

7. The group said they wanted to deal with dependencies, but now that they are, no one is willing to talk about their own dependencies.
   - What can you do to get the discussion moving?
   - What activities/group structures may work here?
   - Is there a place for tutor self-disclosure?
   - When is it not appropriate?

Discussion points and issues raised

- Some of the common difficulties tutors experience include:
  - tutor being seen as expert/therapist/social worker
  - group wanting information, not discussion
  - working with emotions
  - dealing with dominant, talkative women, and quiet women
  - issue of tutor self-disclosure
  - how to open up discussion.
- It is not realistic for tutors to feel they must be experts, especially medical experts: by being an 'expert', others are then 'non-experts'. This may hinder discussion groups using participatory learning methods.

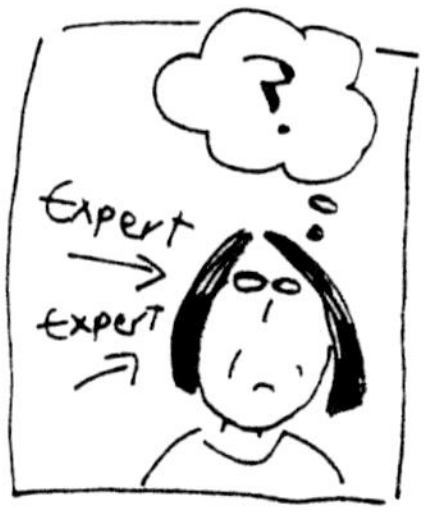

- Tutors/trainers may like to tell the group how they see their role.
- It is possible to bring specialists to talk and to give information about certain subjects. You can also refer women on to local and national agencies and organisations that can give specialist advice and support.
- Tutors can be used and abused by women looking for someone to listen to them. Is it fair to expect the tutor to stay after the session when she may have commitments of her own?
- When groups react negatively to participatory learning methods it can be helpful to acknowledge this and to discuss the relative merits of formal and informal learning methods (see page 33.)
- When tutoring a women's health group, a tutor is not a social worker, therapist, or counsellor. Individuals may have relevant skills in these areas, and may choose to use them, but they are not part of the tutor's role.
- If some women in the group dominate and talk more than others, splitting the group into pairs or small groups may help, especially if there is a clique. If women are quiet, it may have nothing to do with the session; this should be respected.

- Providing a clock and an agenda is a way of getting the group to take responsibility for getting through in time. If time is running short, negotiate quickly with the group about what to focus on.
- When emotions come to the surface, does the tutor have to make everything all right? It may be best to acknowledge the feelings in a straightforward way and not to be immobilised by them. By acknowledging the feelings as important to the women or woman concerned, the group may then begin to share feelings.
- If the group responds with embarrassment, acknowledge this and ask why. This often prompts a wave of relief, followed by discussion about fear of others' emotions and responsibility for making them feel better. Usually our instincts guide us to act in a sensitive way.

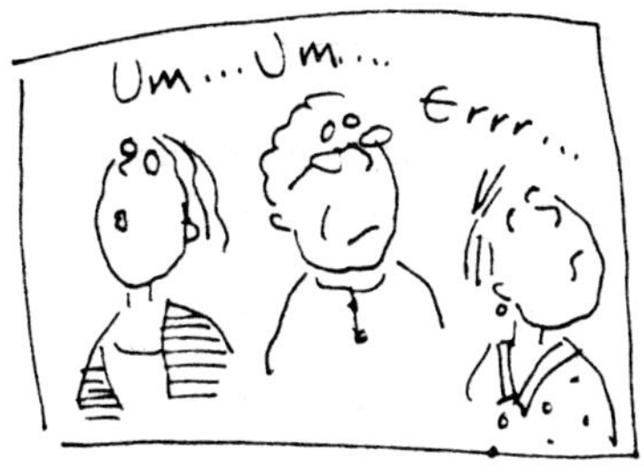

- If it is all too heavy for the group, suggest a tea break, come back, acknowledge, and move on. Later, what has happened can be referred to and feelings can be expressed.
- If energy levels are low, or the subject is depressing, have an enlivener to get the group's energy moving again – a group neck massage, stand up and stretch, and bend or swap seats quickly. (See process activities in section 8.)
- If one woman is feeling down or upset, get the group working and talk to her about what she can do, or ask the group if they have any ideas to offer, or similar experiences.

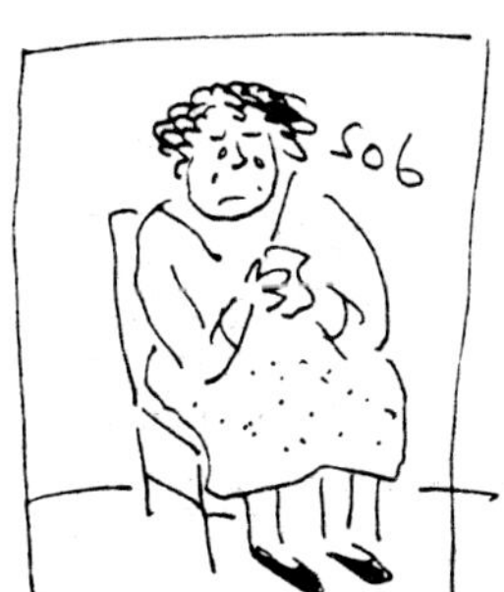

- When should a tutor contribute her own experiences and feelings? It is useful to get a discussion moving around an issue where nobody wants to be seen as different or to be judged. Self-disclosure can set the tone of an activity, and create safe and acceptable boundaries for others.
- The group is not for the tutor. If she feels her emotions will get in the way of responding to the group's needs, it may be worth acknowledging this to the group. Training and support networks can provide this function for tutors and trainers.

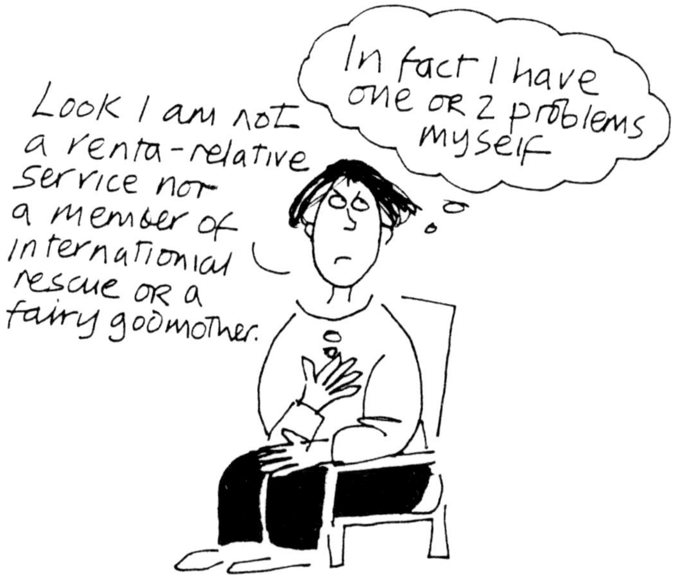
Look I am not a renta-relative service nor a member of international rescue or a fairy godmother.
In fact I have one or 2 problems myself

There are a number of ways of opening up discussions, for example:

- 'What seem to be the three most relevant points to have come up?'
- 'Can someone say what is the single most important issue to them?'
- 'What do you think is the general pattern in all this?'
- 'A lot of ideas – now let's try to find a pattern to it all. Any suggestions?'
- 'Who disagrees? Any other comments to make?'

Each person will develop their own style of tutoring building on individual skills and talents. These styles will differ, and will change through time with experience. (See groupwork activities in section 8.)

Checklist of good practice

Although women will approach groups in different ways, there are elements of good practice that refer to (1) *practicalities* to ensure equality of participation and comfort; (2) *facilitation* to provide boundaries within which learning takes place. Some points may include:

- Arrive early to arrange chairs, organise tea, etc.
- Welcome women as they arrive and provide name labels if needed.
- Explain the agenda and timing. Does anyone have to leave early?
- Clarify tutor role and establish course contract and ground rules.
- Negotiate course content with the group. Be prepared to question aims, to include the group in assessing their relevance and to change tack if needed.
- Have structure and planned activities but be able to be flexible too.
- Keep to the timing, especially for crèche workers.
- Make sure everyone has a chance to contribute.
- Be aware of group structures that can be used to split cliques.
- Leave sufficient time for evaluation.
- Bring group to balanced close.
- Bring women back to real life with ideas for taking things further.

Good practice also can refer to a *code of ethics* for facilitation and tutoring that addresses the issue of tutor responsibility. There are different views about what is the 'right' level of responsibility, for example:

- At one extreme there is the view that the group has responsibility for itself: people choose what is safe within a group situation. The tutor is there only to facilitate communication.
- Alternatively, there is the view that a structured environment is needed for people to feel comfortable enough to be able to make sense of their experiences and to learn. The tutor is responsible for providing the structure and direction.
- Perhaps good working practice involves the tutor taking responsibility for structuring events, and the group also taking a share of the responsibility for the learning that takes place.

It is generally accepted that the tutor/trainer cannot control the group and cannot prepare for every eventuality. Each group is different and the participatory nature of the work leads to unique situations.

Because each group can be different, the tutor should be able to adapt as she goes.

For example:

- using enliveners or fresh-air breaks on the spur of the moment;
- responding to the feel of the group;
- asking why there is little interest in the topic, or why the group can think of nothing to discuss;
- brainstorming on how the group is feeling.
- it is also crucial for tutors and trainers to feel able to challenge a group on attitudes and assumptions. (See page 11.)

Judging success

What counts as success?

In reading manuals and packs, it can seem that to be successful a group needs around 10 or so highly motivated women; when four or five turn up, it can feel a bit of a failure! Yet this is a common occurrence, and the former is a popular misconception. *Women's health education has to start with women wherever they may be.*

So, here is the group and it seems to be doing fine. But how do you know? How do you measure its 'fineness'? Section 7 looks specifically at this issue of *evaluation*; here we look at how evaluation can be used as a tool for self-development.

- Where sessions are intended to be enjoyable and encourage women to participate and interact with each other, then it is possible to sense if things are going well by such things as:
  - a busy hum of voices during a workshop;
  - positive, heated discussions and exchange of views;
  - women staying to chat after the session.
- These sorts of indicators provide a sense of the level, and types, of interactions that are taking place. It can be gratifying to see and hear this group response. You also need to be aware of what is being discussed, to judge whether it is relevant to the aims of the session.

- Other sessions may feel ambiguous – yet the participants say they had a great time and got a lot from it. Because tutors and trainers have different expectations from the participants, and will judge the group differently, it is important to get good, unambiguous participant feedback (see section 8).
- Everyone has awful sessions and agonizes over them. They are part of learning and self-development, which carries on throughout experience. A successful tutor or trainer has the ability to learn from her mistakes and to develop her own style of working.
- There are two main traps to avoid:
  - Doing it all by numbers – following guidelines and manuals like a robot.
  - Using a little skill and relying heavily on strong personality and style – usually acting the comedian!

It is better to understand and feel confident in using skills and learning methods and to adapt them to your own personality and style.

Evaluation as self-development

The main focus of this section has been the importance of learning by making sense of experiences:

- the experience of groups, learning, organising, and working with women;
- using experience to transfer skills from one context to another;
- the collective experience of organising and running events with guidelines and checklists for good practice;
- using your experience to find your own style;
- using the experience of the group to gauge when to alter procedure and do something different.

A cycle of competence has no end-product of the perfect tutor or trainer – simply experienced workers who are learning all the time.

UNCONSCIOUS INCOMPETENCE

unaware you cannot ride a bike

CONSCIOUS INCOMPETENCE

aware you cannot ride it

CONSCIOUS COMPETENCE

riding a bike with total concentration

UNCONSCIOUS COMPETENCE

just doing it and looking at scenery.

Because there are always new situations to grapple with, we return to being aware of not being able to do something. Learning is never-ending.

Information sheet: how people learn

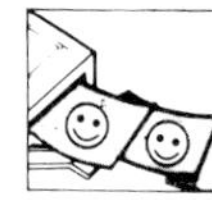

People generally remember:

- 10% of what they read;
- 20% of what they hear;
- 30% of what they see;
- 70% of what they say and write;
- 80% of what they say as they do something.

(*Wiman and Nierhousy*, 1969.)

People generally learn faster when:

- they want to learn;
- social relationships are acknowledged to be important in the learning process;
- there are no distractions;
- there is clarity in communication;
- the content has relevance for the future;
- new information is related to what is already known;
- information is given in a structured way;
- they are able actively to process information, solve problems or practise skills;
- feedback is encouraged;
- the speed of presenting matches the speed of learning.

(*Abbatt and McMahon*, 1987).

Information sheet: the group process

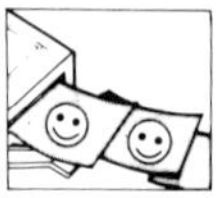

Tuckman has developed a model of group life which highlights five stages the groups go through:

1. Forming
   Anxiety and dependence on leader.
   'What shall we do?'

2. Storming
   Conflict, rebellion against leader.
   'It can't be done.'
   'I won't do it.'

3. Norming
   Development of group cohesion.
   Group norms emerge.
   'We can do it.'

4. Performing
   Doing a task which brings the group together.
   'We are doing it.'

5. Ending
   Desire for group not to end.
   'How can we meet again?'

Many groups progress through these in definite stages, others will jump to and fro from one stage to another.

(from *Working with groups*, Satow & Evans, 1983).

Links with other sections

Section 3: Training in women's health education
Section 4: Working with women
Section 5: Approaching differences between women
Section 7: Evaluation
Section 8: Running sessions/training others
Section 9: Frameworks for women's health training
Section 10: Making it happen – opportunities for training

Resources

See also: General resources section 11
other resources on management/organisation in Resources section 10

Books

Abbatt, F. and McMahon, R. *Teaching health care workers: a practical guide* (1985). Macmillan Education. £4.25.
Although this book is especially aimed at primary health care workers in developing countries, it is a very useful resource which includes learning theory, planning training programmes, and teaching methods.

Bowman, Marion and Norte, M. *Raising money for women: a survivor's guide* (1986). Bedford Square Press. Available from National Council of Voluntary Organisations, 26 Bedford Square, London WC1B 3HU. £5.95.

Buchanan, S. *Replan in rural communities* (1989). NCVO Rural Unit. Available from National Council of Voluntary Organisations, 26 Bedford Square, London WC1B 3HU. £1.
Short report of a one day seminar about the development of education projects with unwaged and unemployed people – raises some useful issues for women working in rural areas.

Community Links. *Ideas annual* (updated annually). Available from Training & Development Unit, Arlewoods Mill, Nursery St, Sheffield. £3.
Innovative ideas and examples of successful groupwork practice.

Sapin, K. and Walters, Geraldine. *Learning from each other: a handbook for participative learning and community work* (1990). Available from William Temple Foundation, Manchester Business School, Manchester M15 6PB. £14.95+p.p.
Practical and flexible handbook, with a wide range of methods for stimulating discussion and including exercises, worksheets and handouts.

Slipman, Sue. *Helping ourselves to power* (1986). Pergamon Press, Oxford. £9.50.
A handbook for women on the skills of public life, including encouraging sections on dealing with fear and very useful exercises to prepare women for negotiating with public bodies, for example, health authorities.

Taylor, Bryce *Experiential learning: a framework for group work skills*. Available from Oasis Publications, Cherry Tree House, Newton-on-Ouse, York. £4.50.

Workers Education Association. *Classes with childcare*. (1982). Available from WEA, 17 Victoria Park Square, Bethnal Green, London E2 4OB. Telephone: 081 983 1515. 50p. Helpful guide for organising childcare.

Workers Education Association. *Health education for women* (1988). Available from WEA North Western District, 4th floor, Crawford House, Precinct Centre, Oxford Road, Manchester M13 9GH. £3.
A useful report and evaluation of women's health education project in WEA North Western District.

Packs

Community Education Training Unit. *Assertion and how to train ourselves*. Available from CETU, Trinity Royd Cottage, Blackwall, Halifax HX1 2EH. £4.65.

Federation of Community Work Training Groups/Association of Metropolitan Authorities. *Learning for action* (1990). Available from FCWTG, 356 Glossop Road, Sheffield S10 2HW. £12.50.
Exploration of courses, learning, sharing and groupwork through examples and exercises.

Organisations

The Open University has published a great deal on every aspect of adult learning and also runs correspondence courses on different issues in community education. Write (well in advance!) to Open University Educational Enterprises Ltd., 12 Cofferidge Close, Stony Stratford, Milton Keynes MK11 1BY.

Referring women on

General resources section 11 gives details of directories of voluntary organisations, charities, self-help groups, and so on.

SECTION SEVEN

Evaluation

	What this section contains	**116**
	How this section can be of use	**117**
	What is evaluation?	**118**
	The process of evaluation	120
	Why evaluate?	
7.1	ACTIVITY: why evaluate?	121
7.2	ACTIVITY: feelings about evaluation	123
	Who is the evaluation for?	**125**
	What to evaluate?	**125**
	Who should evaluate?	**126**
	When to evaluate	**127**
	How to evaluate	
7.3	ACTIVITY: how to evaluate a women's health event	127
	Evaluation by participants of women's health events	128
	Possible responses to different methods of evaluation by participants	129
	Evaluating yourself as a tutor/trainer	131
	What to do with the evaluation	**132**
	Links with other sections	**132**
	Resources	**133**

'My training day was a great success', you say. 'Ten women turned up.' But you had expected 20. And of the 10 who did come, three left at lunch time, and of the seven remaining, none returned the evaluation sheet you gave out at the end of the day.

You judge your women's health course to have been a success. After all, you had 15 women on the register at the first meeting. But didn't several women drop out along the way (you're not sure why); and at the end, had you achieved what you'd set out to do at the beginning?

Too often evaluation is seen in terms of statistics: how many women came to your course or training event, which minority ethnic groups you attracted, how many older women came, and so on. But to monitor and evaluate effectively, you need more than the numbers game: you need to decide at the initial planning stage what aspects of the work you want to evaluate. There are three key aspects – the process, the output and the outcome.

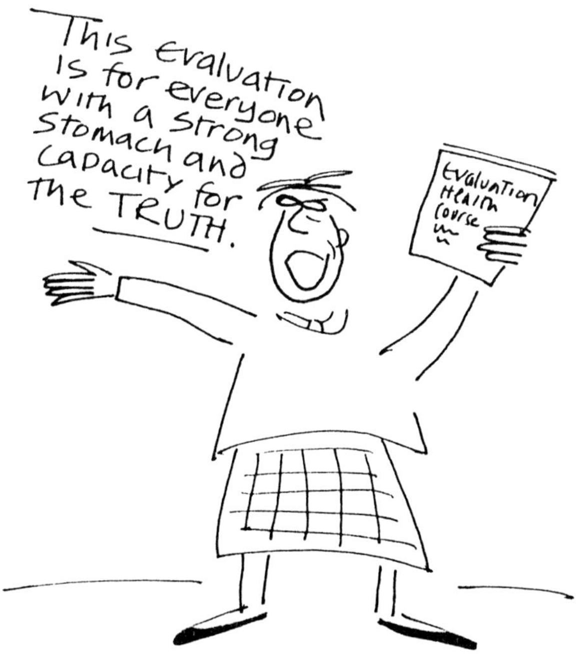
This evaluation is for everyone with a strong stomach and capacity for the TRUTH.
Evaluation Health Course

What this section contains

This section follows on from self-development in Section 6. It:

- explains what evaluation is;
- provides activities for looking at why, and how, and what to evaluate;
- considers who should evaluate and when to evaluate;
- gives possible outcomes from different types of participant evaluation;
- suggests how to evaluate yourself as a tutor/trainer;
- offers ideas for what to do with your evaluation.

How this section can be of use

This section may:

- give you some ideas on how to evaluate;
- help you appraise your own practice of evaluation;
- be useful background reading to the participants' evaluation activities in Section 8;
- be a basis for running a training session/event around the issue of evaluation;
- prompt you to provide your own evaluation materials.

What is evaluation?

Evaluation can seem like a burden imposed by others when other work is so pressing and time is short. The prospect of asking yourself searching questions about your own practice may be threatening, and because evaluation is often associated with formal research methods you may feel you don't know how to evaluate effectively.

> Good evaluation assesses what has been achieved against what was intended and explains why this has happened, in order to derive some lessons for future work. It is about measuring change and making changes to approach more nearly the core purpose of the work. (Graessle & Kingsley, 1986.)

One of the most important aims of evaluation is to *assess what is being achieved against what was intended*. In women's health education this is not always simple, for example, let us look at a women's health course:

Aims

- To encourage women to stop smoking.

Objectives

1. To lead to at least 40% of women stopping smoking completely during the course, and 25% of women being non-smokers three months after the end of the course.
2. To increase participants' awareness of the risks of smoking, the reasons why women smoke, and the problems associated with stopping smoking.

Evaluation

Such a course could be evaluated using both quantitative and qualitative methods. *Quantitative* evaluation has close links with both epidemiological and medical research. (Epidemiology is the statistical analysis of health and illness in large populations.)

To make a quantitative evaluation of objective (1) of the women's health course above, you would need to:

- find out how many participants smoked at the beginning of the course;
- monitor how many women stopped smoking completely during the course;
- follow up women three months after the course to see how many were still non-smokers.

To make a quantitative evaluation of objective (2), you would need to:

- Find out at the beginning of the course what women know about the risks of smoking, why they thought they smoked, and the problems they anticipate in giving up smoking.
- Measure at the end of the course women's knowledge of the links between smoking and health problems, awareness of their reasons for smoking, and the problems associated with stopping smoking.

But quantitative methods alone lead to partial evaluation. Qualitative evaluation can lead to a better overall picture gained by including women's views and feelings.

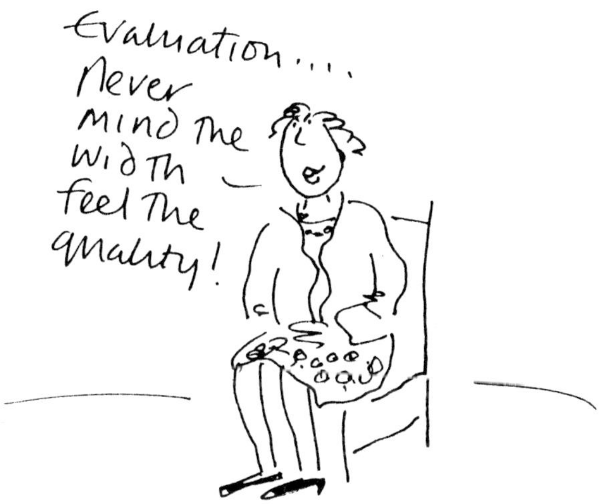

Qualitative methods are firmly rooted in the community development approach, and are finding their way into community health, adult and health education, and a growing body of feminist research. Evaluation in this tradition

> is intended to help those involved look at what has happened, to assess what was valuable and to suggest what to build on. It is an approach which aims to recognise that clients and their perspectives are central not only in the work itself but also in reflection on the work and making necessary changes.
>
> (Graessle & Kingsley, 1986).

A qualitative evaluation of the women's health course above could enhance the quantitative evaluation (i.e. how many women stopped smoking) by showing how women had developed a better understanding of why they find it difficult to change their smoking behaviour, what areas of the course women learned most from, what they valued most, and how it was most relevant to their lives.

Thus evaluation is often enhanced by using a combination of both *quantitative* (how many women came to the course? what measurable changes happened as a result of their attendance?) and *qualitative* methods (what did women feel about the course? what effects did they think it might have had on their behaviour?).

The process of evaluation

Evaluation is a process of reflection, appraisal, change, and building on experience. It involves the following stages:

1. *Assessing* needs.
2. *Assessing* available resources.
3. *Establishing* clear aims.
4. *Developing* objectives (activities or services) to meet these aims.
5. *Planning* activities or services.
6. *Collecting* data about what you are doing, while you are doing it.
7. *Reviewing* what you have done, to see if you are doing what you set out to do.
8. *Evaluating* what you have done, to see if needs have been met and aims fulfilled.
9. *Learning* from the experience and applying what you have learned to future work.

For diagrammatic form see opposite.

The following questions may help to make evaluation a manageable and logical process:

- WHY evaluate?
- WHO is the evaluation for?
- WHAT to evaluate?
- WHEN to evaluate?
- WHO should evaluate?
- HOW to evaluate?
- WHAT TO DO with the evaluation?

Process of Evaluation

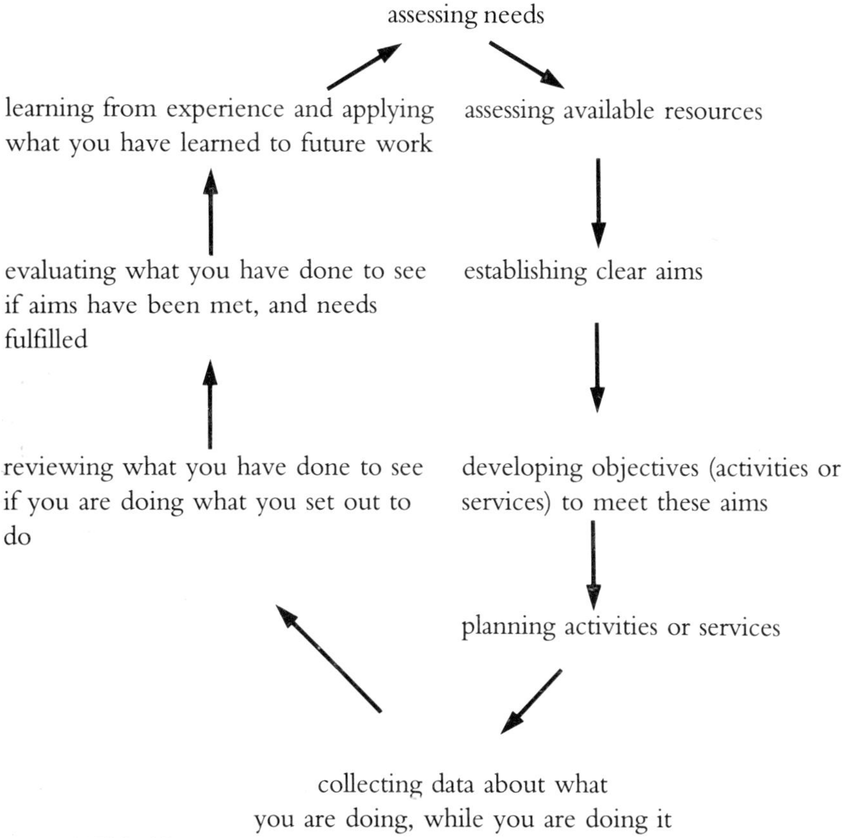

(Adapted from Sandy Merrit, 1988.)

Why evaluate?

7.1 ACTIVITY: why evaluate?

Aims

- To share reasons for the importance of evaluation.

Materials

Flipchart and markers.

Method **Time: 30 minutes**

1. Ask the question 'I think it is important to evaluate because . . .'
2. Flipchart responses.

Discussion points and issues raised
Responses may depend on:

- who is doing the exercise
  - workers may resent having to justify their existence to funders/employers/managers (who are rightly interested in value-for-money);
- previous experience of evaluation
  - if you see the purpose of evaluation as merely to placate funders or managers rather than for your own benefit, then you may place less importance on evaluation;
- acknowledgement of the need to evaluate yourself to measure what is being done and ways of improving.

The importance of evaluation, then, is to:

- Clarify aims and objectives.
- See if we are meeting these.
- See whether we are making the best use of ourselves as a resource.
- Measure the suitability of course/event content and effectiveness of materials.
- Assess the adequacy of the organisational arrangements.
- Assess process as well as outcome.
- Be accountable to ourselves, our colleagues, funders, employers, and participants.
- Judge cost, time, and effectiveness.
- Assess whether original needs are being met.
- Generate change and improve ways of working.
- Work towards models of good practice.
- Share our experience.
- Demonstrate effectiveness in order to secure continuing support and funding.

7.2 ACTIVITY: feelings about evaluation

Aims

- To explore feelings about evaluation.

Materials

Flipchart and markers.

Method **Time: 45 minutes**

1. In small groups, hand out two flipchart sheets to each group, one headed 'negative' and the other 'positive'.
2. Each group writes their anxieties about evaluation on the 'negative' flipchart, and the things that excite them on the 'positive' flipchart.
3. When finished, exchange flipcharts between groups and compare.

Possible responses (from evaluation workshop with community health workers and health authority officers)

Anxieties (negative)

- Time.
- Truth.
- Aims and objectives lacking clarity.
- Resentment.
- Cuts in funding.
- Knowing how/where to start.
- Fear of showing that you are not achieving your aims.
- Conflict between funding body's and workers' expectations.
- How to make results credible to funding body.
- How does evaluation fit in with the philosophy of what you are doing?
- Feeling the need for one evaluation report for funders and one for workers.

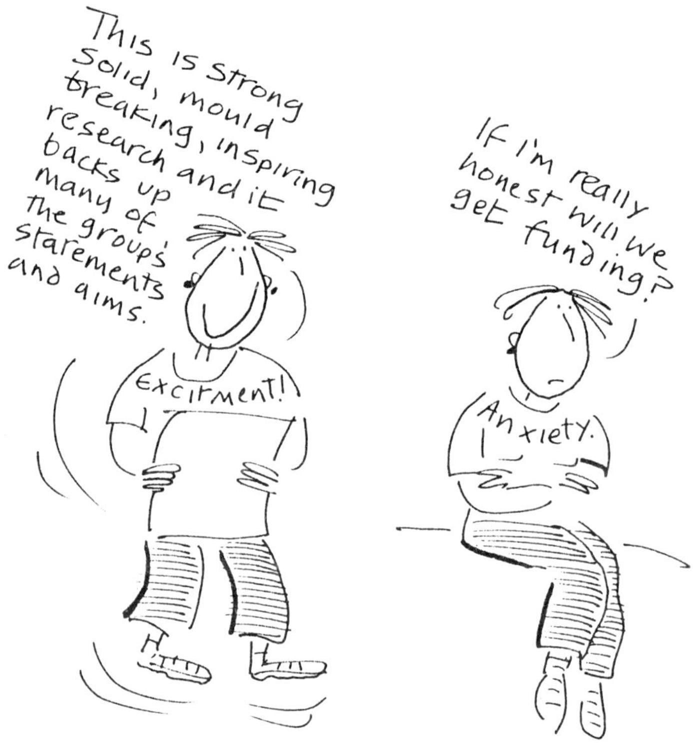
This is strong solid, mould breaking, inspiring research and it backs up many of the groups' statements and aims.
Excitment!
If I'm really honest will we get funding?
Anxiety.

Excitement (positive)

- New ideas
- Favourable outcome, co-operation from funders.
- Involvement.
- Learning to improve your own work.
- Focuses aims.
- Feedback.
- Information to promote work/funding.
- Public accountability.
- Positive feedback from participants.
- Constructive criticism.
- Confidence-boosting.

- Find out how you are doing.
- Self-development.

Who is the evaluation for?

Defining who we are evaluating for will determine what we evaluate.

Funders and employers may particularly want to know that goals have been achieved, that the work is cost-effective, how the work can lead to policy change, or ensure the future of similar work.

Trainers will want to know the above, plus they may want to assess teamwork, practice, and job satisfaction.

Participants need to be given the opportunity to reflect on their experience of participating in health education (or using a service/provision) to assess whether their needs are being met.

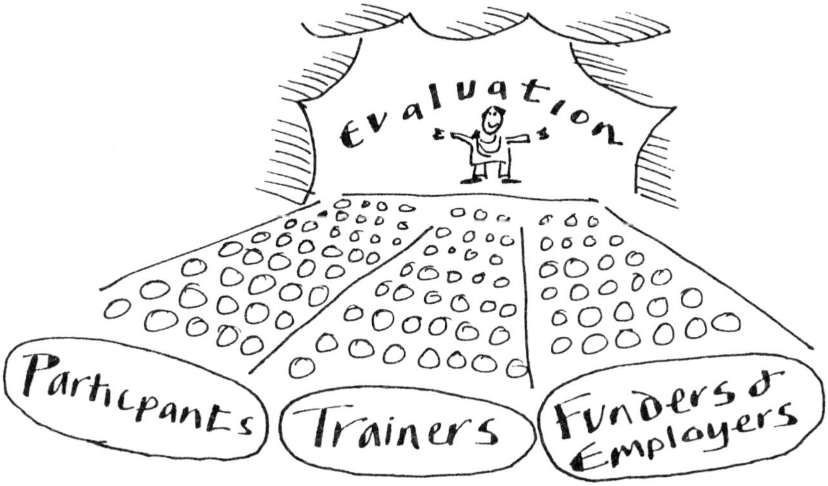

What to evaluate?

Whoever you are evaluating for, it will be necessary to evaluate the *process*, the *output*, and the *outcome*. This involves looking at your original objectives for the event, and considering whether or not you met them.

- *The process* involves looking at the planning and running of the event. You will want to look at the actual programme, and the learning methods used. You may also consider the venue, the crèche and the refreshments. You could evaluate the process through *self evaluation* (e.g. by asking yourself how you did, if there was anything you were dissatisfied with, how you could improve next time, see page 131) and through *participant evaluation* (getting feedback from participants, see page 128).

- *The output* will include any reports, articles, publications, seminars, and so on done as a result of your work.
- *The outcome* is achieved by evaluating the effect of your work on women's health. This can be done through assessing:
  changes in knowledge (interviews/discussions/observation/written questionnaires);
  changes in attitudes (observing changes during and after health education activity/scales which ask participants to rate their attitudes and values, etc.);
  changes in skills (observing how participants demonstrate a newly acquired skill);
  decision making (noting what participants say they intend to do);
  behaviour change (observing behaviour of individuals and groups/demonstration of new behaviour/record of behaviour – numbers attending, say, a family planning clinic or participant keeping her own diary of behaviour).

(See also the evaluation activities for participants in section 8.)

Process, output, and *outcome* can all be measured via *quantitative* methods or *qualitative* methods, or a combination of both.

Who should evaluate?

> If the evaluation is to be a tool for change, rather than merely a measure of change, then the way it is set up and who does it are crucial. The more people involved in evaluation, the greater commitment to its outcome.
>
> (Graessle & Kingsley, 1986.)

There may be opportunities to contract-in an expert to evaluate your work. Advantages are that an 'outsider' will be objective, have time, and may have more knowledge of research methods. Evaluation, however, is a vehicle whereby *people on all levels can be involved*, ranging from management to participants.

The evaluation of women's health courses/training is a two-way process:

- For the *tutor/group leader*, evaluation provides a means for assessing:
  – level of individual participation;

- relevance of the course content;
- success of different teaching methods;
- extent of development of group cohesion;
- direction the group is moving in;
- successes and failures of the course/event;
- own skills and effectiveness.

- For the *group members/participants* evaluation, can:
  - improve the relevance and quality of the course/event;
  - encourage them to have control over, and participate in, their own learning process;
  - enable reflection on learning and personal development.

When to evaluate

To be effective, evaluation should be ongoing and part of usual practice. When planning an event and deciding objectives, it is useful to decide how you will evaluate them; while running events, you will need to monitor and review.

Monitoring, involves keeping records of events as they are occurring. This requires careful thinking about what you want to record. Monitoring however, is not an end in itself.

Reviewing – stopping and reflecting at regular intervals – is important during an event as well as after a number of events. You may, for example, want to take stock halfway through a day event, or you may want to show how many courses or groups you have run in a certain period, how many attended, which succeeded, and which failed.

Both monitoring and reviewing provide information that is essential to an effective evaluation.

How to evaluate

7.3 ACTIVITY: How to evaluate a women's health event

Aims

- To share the different ways of evaluating.

Materials
Flipchart and markers.

Method **Time: 40 minutes**

1. Brainstorm the different ways of evaluating.
2. Flipchart responses.
3. In large group, discuss the advantages and disadvantages of each.

Possible responses

- Evaluation by participants at end of session:
  - verbally;
  - written (evaluation sheet, Post-its, tick symbols);
  - guided fantasy through session.
- Evaluation by questionnaire completed after event and returned.
- Evaluation by participant follow-up:
  - phone call soon after event;
  - follow-up session to discuss event and move forward.
- Evaluation of yourself as group leader/tutor:
  - feedback from participants;
  - reflection on content, process, timing;
  - colleague sits in and gives feedback later;
  - discuss with co-tutor after;
  - write up session/event and circulate to others doing similar work for their comments.

Evaluation by participants of women's health course or training event

There are many different ways of finding out what the participants felt (see evaluation activities in section 8). Which ones you choose will depend on such things as:

- Participants' literacy and language levels.
- The length and type of event, for example: a detailed questionnaire given out at the end of a one-off, two-hour session with a group you have never met before probably will not be answered; a long-term or residential event will give you scope for choosing a detailed questionnaire.
- If expectations have been written up and displayed on a flipchart at the beginning of the event, women can then refer to these to see if they have been met.

Possible responses to different methods of evaluation by participants

Ways of evaluating at the end of an event.

- Verbal feedback (in round or small groups)
  Advantages
  – group members hear what everyone thinks;
  – tutor gets to hear (written evaluation sheets do not all get returned);
  – verbal feedback gets round literacy difficulties.
  Disadvantages
  – women may feel unable to be critical or negative.

- Written feedback (questionnaire)
  Questionnaires should be clear, and open to systematic interpretation and recording of respones. Using numbers 1–4 ('best' to 'worst') to ring for each question is quick and efficient.
  Advantages
  – anonymity (women may be afraid to be verbally critical).
  Disadvantages
  – time: women may have to leave so responses may be hurried and not thought out (if you want evaluation sheets filled in at the event, do not make them long);
  – fixed questions means you will only get comments on issues addressed in the questionnaire. A final question such as 'any other comments?' gives an opportunity to raise other issues.

- Other written feedback, for example Post-its
  Advantages
  – quick;
  – perhaps less threatening than questionnaires (can be pictures, symbols).
  Disadvantages
  – you do not get as much feedback as from questionnaires.

- Guided fantasy (see page 159)
  Advantages
  – women are able to reflect for themselves on what they have gained.
  Disadvantages
  – no one else knows.

Ways of evaluating subsequent to event

- Evaluation sheet given out at the end of an event to take away, complete and return (questionnaire, sentence-completion sheets).

Advantages
- enables scope for more detail, since women will not be pressed for time or be tired as they could be at the end of an event;
- reflection after an event can lead to more fruitful evaluation;
- after a specific event women can be clearer about how they would like to move forward;
- questions can have 'other comments' as well as numbers to circle for each question, allowing for increased feedback;
- open-ended questions allow for a diversity of responses.

Disadvantages
- however well-meaning women are, you will not receive back all evaluation sheets (including a stamped addressed envelope often helps return rates!);
- open-ended questions, or sentence-completion sheets, are more difficult to collate (but very worthwhile if you do).

● Follow-up phone call

Advantages
- distance often allows for greater clarity of feelings;
- participants will feel their views are valued.

Disadvantages
- not all women will feel able to be frank or critical, and may therefore resent the phone call;
- time-consuming and costly.

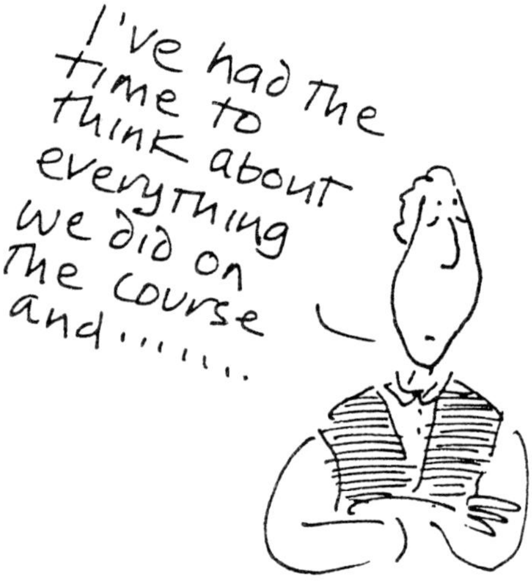
I've had the time to think about everything we did on the course and.......

- Follow-up meeting
  Advantages
  – distance from event often enables clarity of feelings;
  – encourages discussion about 'where to next?'
  Disadvantages
  – only small percentage of original participants will come;
  – needs organisation, venue, etc.;
  – time-consuming.

Evaluating yourself as a tutor/trainer

By evaluating what participants felt about the event, you will have some idea of how you are doing. In order to evaluate your own work, however, you need to monitor in other ways as well:

(1) A standard form to fill in for each event you run will give you a lot of information about each event, and will enable you to compare events, in order to draw out models of good practice. Filling in a form also disciplines you to commit to paper the facts and impressions that were fresh in your mind at the time, but get lost afterwards. The form might include such questions as:

- Who came? Did it attract the women you were hoping to reach? If not, why not?
- How did the women who came hear about it?
- Was the venue easy to find, accessible for women with disabilities, prams, and so on? Was it comfortable?
- Was the childcare good?
- Was the course content or programme okay?
- Were the teaching approaches and methods appropriate?
- If they did the course again, what would participants change?
- What did participants gain from the event?
- How did the course differ from participants' expectations?
- What would they like to do after the event?

(2) Having a colleague to sit in with you during a session can be extremely useful for honest feedback. Key criteria need to be decided upon beforehand. To reciprocate you could offer to sit in on one of her events.

(3) Writing up the event and circulating it to others for their comments can give you valuable feedback. It also encourages you to be really clear about how to write up the event, which can only be to your advantage. You could offer to comment on others' events in the same way.

What to do with the evaluation

Evaluation can improve practice, influence planning and decision making, provide information, and produce models of good practice. It also can be boring, inaccessible, and an academic exercise for funders that does no more than gather dust. To ensure it is not simply an end in itself, thought should be given as to how the evaluation is presented, and how it can be used.

If the evaluation is for funders, it need not be a dry, formal report. A presentation meeting may be more appropriate, and will give the funders a chance to ask questions – and the evaluators a chance to find out if the funders were clear about the aims in the first place. Funders should take the responsibility for negotiating realistic aims for the work at the start and how these might be evaluated.

It is important to feed back your evaluation to the women who participated in the work. Think of imaginative ways of doing this, either in person or through a lively report.

Think about circulating your evaluation report not just to colleagues, employers, and funders, but wider, both locally and nationally, to:

- sympathetic media (local rag, radio);
- local and national women's health networks;
- local community health council and other community organisations;
- local health promotion unit.

By effectively evaluating what we do, and by circulating and sharing the results, we can learn from each other.

Links with other sections

Section 1: About this handbook

Section 6: Learning from experience

Section 8: Running sessions/training others: Activities for participant evaluation (evaluation round, guided fantasy, small groups, post-its, 'one thing I am taking away with me', sample evaluation sheets)

Evaluation sheet to give feedback on this handbook (pages 323–327).

Resources

Books

Ball, Mog. *Evaluation in the voluntary sector* (1988). Available from Forbes Trust, Forbes House, 9 Artillery Lane, London E1 7LP. Telephone: 071-377 8484. £4.95.
Mainly theoretical account, although with some useful examples – this would make good reading for groups hoping to apply for funding. The Forbes Trust have published a range of papers and conference proceedings on evaluation in the voluntary sector.

Edwards, J. *Evaluation: a practical handbook for teachers and organisers* (1991). WEA. Available from WEA, W. Lancs and Cheshire District, 7/8 Bluecoat Chambers, School Lane, Liverpool L1 3BX. Tel: 051 709 8023. £10.
Includes evaluating yourself, your course, your institution, and evaluation methods.

Feek, Warren. *Working effectively: a guide to evaluation techniques*. Bedford Square Press. £4.95.
Includes a range of exercises for evaluation which could be explored in groups.

Graessle, Lois and Kingsley, Sue. *Measuring change and making changes – an approach to evaluation* (1986). London Community Health Resource. Available from NCHR, 57 Chalton Street, London NW1 1HU. £3.25.
Highlights and discusses evaluating health in the community, with a comprehensive bibliography.

Hedley, Rodney. *Measuring success – a guide to evaluation for voluntary and community groups* (1985). Neighbourhood Care Action Programme. Available from Advance, 14 Bloomsbury Square, London WC1 £3.

Meadows, Ann and Turkie, Alan. (ed. Paul Hodson) *How are we doing?* (1988). Bedford Square Press, London.
An introduction to self-evaluation for voluntary groups.

Merritt, S. Getting it right: monitoring and evaluation in community jobs. LVSC. *Voluntary Voice*, March 1988, issue no. 23.

NCHR. *Bibliography no. 2: evaluation* (1991). Available from National Community Health Resource, 57 Chalton St., London NW1 1HU. Telephone: 071 383 3841. £3.95.

North Manchester Health Promotion Unit. *Self-help guide to evaluation* (October 1986). Available from North Manchester Health Promotion Unit, Beech Mount, Harpurhey, Manchester M9 1XG.

Pollitt, Christopher. *Evaluation of community health projects in Walker, North Kenton and Riverside* (1989). Available from Riverside Child Health Project, Atkinson Road Clinic, Atkinson Road, Benwell, Newcastle upon Tyne.

Turner, Leslie and Willis, Elaine. *Measuring up: guidelines on the self-evaluation of volunteer projects* (1987). Up to 12 copies free from Volunteer Centre, 29 Lower Kings Road, Berkhamsted, Herts HP4 2AB.
Pamphlet aimed at organisations employing volunteers, with some useful general guidelines on evaluation.

WEA North Western District. *Health education for women: a report and evaluation of work in WEA North Western District* (1988). Available from WEA, 4th Floor, Crawford House, Precinct Centre, Oxford Road, Manchester M13 9GH. Telephone: 061 273 7652. £3.

Packs
Women learning together – training materials and guidelines for tutors (1988). Available from Salford Women's Education Forum, Education Office, Chapel Street, Salford M3 5LT. £2.
This is a course to develop skills in running women's education courses and groups.

Working towards change – a Workers Education Association training pack for tutors in women's education (1986). Available from WEA, 17 Victoria Park Square, Bethnal Green, London E2 9PB. Telephone: 081 983 1515. £5.95.

Newsletters
Community health action (Issue 12 Spring 1989). Available from NCHR, 57 Chalton Street, London NW1 1HU. Telephone: 071 383 3841.
This is the newsletter of the National Community Health Resource. It is a special issue on evaluating community health projects, with articles on evaluation, publications, resources and where to seek help.

SECTION EIGHT

Running sessions/training others

What this section contains **136**
How this section can be of use **136**
Process-based activities
Introductions/icebreakers 137
Expectations 142
Promoting trust 145
Mood lighteners/enliveners 149
Evaluation 156
Closing 163
Adapting a teaching method for different topics
Contraception game 171
Exploring dependencies/addictions game 173
Stress game 175
Safer-sex game 176
Activities for training others
Acknowledging and building on existing skills 178
Groupwork 184
Planning events 201
Clarifying/strategising 209
Networking 214
Support 222
Links with other sections **225**
Resources **225**

What this section contains

If you are a tutor who is running women's health sessions or courses, this section shows you how, with a few extra skills, *you can train others* to run women's health sessions and courses.

Many different kinds of *activities* are included:

- process-based activities to use if you are running health sessions or training others to do the same;
- activities to show how one learning/teaching method can be adapted to suit many topics;
- activities to use in training women to run women's health sessions.

How this section can be of use

- If you are thinking of *running women's health sessions.*
- If you are a *women's health tutor*, it may
  - give you ideas, methods, and activities;
  - reaffirm what you are already doing;
  - provide you with materials;
  - give you confidence in training others to run women's health sessions.
- If you are a *trainer*, it may
  - give you new ideas, methods, and activities;
  - be useful for evaluating your own practice;
  - offer activities that can be adapted to suit your own needs;
  - give you groupwork activities for training around groupwork skills.
- If you are a *self-help group*, you could use the methods and activities for yourselves.
- If you work in *adult education*, you may want to consider using women's health as a training tool.
- Activities around *networking and support* may be useful in whatever work you are doing.

Activities

Women's health sessions can range from a two-hour event to a course that extends over weeks or months. They can involve *tutoring* women in women's health issues or topics, or *training others* to tutor around women's health. Whether long or short, tutoring or training, all sessions have a beginning, a middle, and an end, and they all use process activities to make them happen:

- first, women need to get to know each other (introductions/icebreakers, page 137);
- even if you know what women would like to do, asking them at the beginning is important (expectations, page 142);
- if women are to work together trust must be established by agreeing guidelines for working together (promoting trust activities, page, 145);
- when a group gets tired and bogged down, it will need a change of pace and direction (mood lighteners/enliveners, page 149);
- at the end of a session, it is useful for you and the group to know how everyone feels (evaluation activities, page 156).
- it may be necessary to end on a positive note after a lot of emotions have been shared, or, if group cohesion is needed, to round off the session. (See structuring sessions in sections 6 and 9; closing activities, page 163.)

Process-based activities

Introductions/icebreakers

8.1 ACTIVITY: names

Aims
- To enable women to begin to know each other.

Materials

Two large flipchart sheets on floor, and two thick marker pens.

Method **Time: 10 minutes**

1. Ask each woman in turn to write down her name on the flipchart sheets, and say something about her name.

Possible outcomes

- Women can say as much or as little as they like.
- Often leads to laughter.
- It can be difficult for women with a mobility impairment to get down on their knees and write (something to be aware of).

8.2 ACTIVITY: ballgame

Aims

- To help women to learn each others' names, or to remind each other at a later point in the session/event.

Materials

One small soft ball.

Method **Time: 5 minutes**

1. Ask women to sit in a circle.
2. Ask each woman in turn to say who they are.
3. Throw the ball to a woman, saying her name as you do so.
4. She in turn throws the ball to another woman, naming her.
5. Continue until you think everyone is becoming clear on each others' names.

8.3 ACTIVITY: paired introductions

Aims

- To begin to share with each other and listen carefully.

Materials

None

Method **Time: 15–20 minutes**

1. Ask women to sit in a circle.
2. Ask each woman to talk about herself for five minutes to the woman on her right (if there is an odd number, make a threesome).
3. Ask each woman to introduce her partner to the large group (e.g. 'This is Jaswinda, she lives in Manchester, she is involved in . . .').

8.4 ACTIVITY: handshakes

Aims
- To move about, talk, and get to know each other.

Materials
Paper and pens.

Method **Time: 10 minutes**

1. Give out paper and pens.
2. Ask each woman to write her name and then put her paper on the floor in front of her, facing out.
3. Go round the group, each woman saying her name in turn.
4. Collect papers and hand out at random.
5. Each woman finds the person whose name she has, shakes hands, and says something positive she has noticed about her.

Possible outcomes
- May take time as women are both seeking and being sought by each other.

8.5 ACTIVITY: fantasy introductions

Aims
- To help group members to get to know each other.
- To lessen feelings of difference and status within the group.
- To reduce anxiety about how much to tell others.

Materials
None

Method **Time: 25 minutes**

1. Ask each woman to reflect on what she would like to share about a fantasy life she would like to lead.
2. Ask women to pair up and share for five minutes whatever they feel comfortable with. Explain that they will be introducing each other to the large group.
3. Bring women back to the main group. Allow each woman one minute to introduce her partner.
4. Allow a few minutes to talk about the fantasies.
5. Ask each woman to say who she really is, and what her interest in the event is.

Possible outcomes

- Appropriate for day-workshops or ongoing courses where time is available for grounding women in their real lives.
- It may be necessary to be directive about moving on.
- There may need to be time at the end to discuss what came up, for example, what does this say about our lives, self-images, choices we make. Although this will take time, it will enable the working-through of feelings.
- Some women find it hard to think of fantasies. It is important to recognise this and to change the activity if someone is uncomfortable.
- Can also be used as a mood lightener/enlivener.

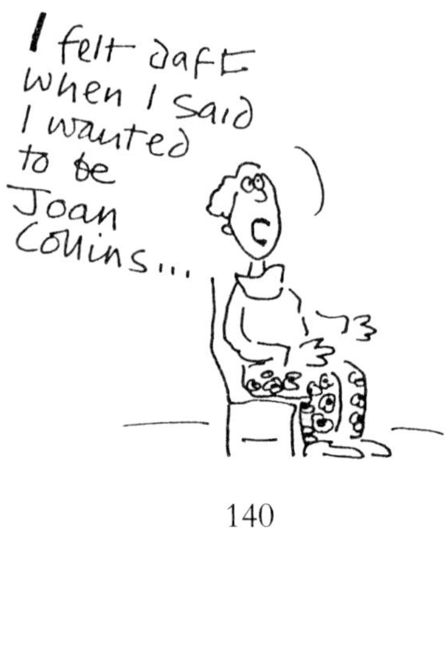
I felt daft when I said I wanted to be Joan Collins...

8.6 ACTIVITY: telling the truth

Aims

- To begin to work together in small groups.
- To start to break down barriers.
- To have fun!

Materials

Paper and pens.

Method **Time: 15 minutes**

1. Divide into small groups.
2. Ask each woman to write down three things about herself – one false and two true.
3. One woman reads out her statement.
4. The group asks questions to discover the false statement, for example by asking factual questions to see if they can be answered, or by checking if answers are consistent.
5. The group collectively decides which is the false statement, which the woman confirms.

Possible outcomes

- Surprise, laughter, fun!

8.7 ACTIVITY: what I wanted to be when I grew up

Aims

- To break the ice and lighten the atmosphere.
- To think more creatively and imaginatively.
- To reduce all women to the same level.

Materials

None

Method **Time: 10 minutes**

1. Ask women to sit in a circle.
2. Each woman says in turn what she wanted to be when she grew up.

Possible outcomes

- Some women may find this difficult if they think they will be judged; best done with a group that knows each other.

Variation

Can be used as an icebreaker or mood lightener:
Ask women to say what . . . 'If I was a tree/flower/animal . . .'; 'If I won the pools . . .'; 'If I was re-incarnated as a film star I would be . . .'; and why.

Expectations

8.8 ACTIVITY: round

Aims

- To find out what women want from the event.
- To share expectations.
- To let the tutor see if the planned programme will meet women's expectations.

Materials

Flipchart and pens.

Method **Time: 10 minutes**

1. Ask women to sit in a circle.
2. Each woman to say in turn what she would like from the day. Flipchart responses.
3. Display flipchart for the rest of the event.

Possible outcomes

- If women have unrealistic expectations, say what is possible to achieve and what is not. If publicity has been clear then expectations should be realistic.

8.9 ACTIVITY: index cards

Aims

- To find out what women want from the event.
- To share expectations.
- To let the tutor see if the planned programme will meet women's expectations.

Materials

Index cards, pens, and bin/box/bag.

Method **Time: 10 minutes**

1. Give each woman a card.
2. Ask her to write down what she would like from the day, stressing that what she writes will be anonymous, but will be shared with the group.
3. Collect all cards in the bin/box/bag.
4. Take cards out, blank-side-up, and shuffle.
5. Each woman takes a card (if she picks her own, replace with another).
6. Women in turn read out what is on the card.
7. Flipchart responses.

Possible outcomes

- Less confident women may be more specific about their needs if they can express them anonymously rather than verbally to the whole group.

8.10 ACTIVITY: what I want from this event

Aims

- To help women to clarify their expectations for themselves.

Materials

Worksheet (page 144) for each woman.

(continued on page 145)

WORKSHEET: what I want from this event

A8.10

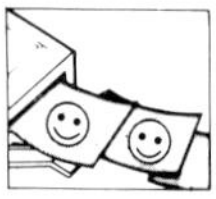

Fill in three things under each of the following headings:

In this event I want . . .

In this event I do not want . . .

I wish I knew more about . . .

I wish I knew better how to . . .

(Adapted from WEA North of Scotland, *Getting Started*.)

Method **Time: 20–30 minutes**

1. Ask women, individually, in pairs, or small groups, to fill in the Worksheet.
2. Feed back to large group. Flipchart responses.
3. Work out similarities. Flipchart clusters that women are interested in.

Possible outcomes

- Some women may find it easier to say what they do not want than what they do want.
- You will get a better idea of what women want than if you ask them what they would like to do.
- Useful for a series of sessions or a course. For a short one-off session or a one-day event the programme will be less flexible.

Promoting trust

8.11 ACTIVITY: ground rules I

Aims
- To agree guidelines for working together.

Materials
Flipchart, pens.

Method **Time: 10 minutes**

1. Ask women to sit in a circle.
2. Brainstorm ways that would enable the group to work together effectively. Flipchart responses.
3. You may need to prompt. Ask women to think of other experiences they have had in groups:
   - what they did/did not like about the group;
   - what made them feel comfortable/uncomfortable.

4. Check that everyone agrees. Point out that the group is responsible for ensuring that the ground rules are adhered to. Are there any additional responsibilities they would like you as tutor to agree to?
5. Display the ground rules for the rest of the event. Stress that the group can add more rules if necessary during the event.

Variation
In pairs, ask women to think about how they would like to work together as a group. Discuss in large group and flipchart.

Possible outcomes
A list might include:

- confidentiality;
- listening as well as talking;
- respecting others' opinions;
- acknowledging different levels of knowledge and experience;
- no one forced to contribute;
- keeping to time;
- no smoking in agreed areas.

8.12 ACTIVITY: ground rules II – brick wall

Aims
- To agree guidelines for working together.

Materials
A5 pieces of coloured paper (10 for each group), markers, an enormous sheet of paper for 'brick wall' (sellotape 6 flipchart sheets together), and glue.

Method **Time: 30–35 minutes**

1. Divide women into small groups.
2. Give each group 10 pieces of coloured paper ('bricks') and markers.
3. Write a ground rule or guideline on each 'brick'.

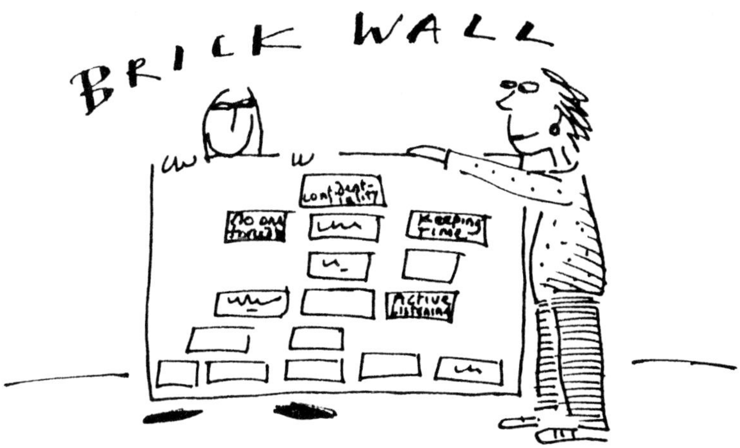

4. When finished, ask a group for one of their 'bricks' and read it out. Ask if other groups have a similar 'brick'.
5. Place these together horizontally on the 'wall'.
6. Continue until all 'bricks' have been discussed.
7. The ground rules that have been agreed by the group are stuck to the 'wall', which is then displayed for the rest of the event.

Possible outcomes

- Several 'bricks' on the same theme will show the importance of this particular ground rule to the group.

(Thanks to Stockport Health Promotion Unit.)

★ 8.13 ACTIVITY: things you never knew about me

Aims

- To encourage women to feel comfortable about sharing personal information.

Materials

Flipchart paper, markers.

Method **Time: 10 minutes**

1. Divide women into pairs and give each pair paper and markers.

2. One woman tells the other 'Five things you never knew about me', who writes them down.
3. Change places.
4. Put finished flipcharts on wall to be looked at during next break.

(Thanks to Greta Wilson.)

★ 8.14 ACTIVITY: trust me . . .

Aims

- To enable women to trust each other through touch.

Materials

None.

Method **Time: 10 minutes**

1. Divide women into pairs.
2. One woman closes her eyes or puts on a blindfold.
3. The other woman leads her slowly around the room, while the 'blind' woman asks if she is near an object, in danger, and so on.
4. Change places.

Possible outcomes

- Some women are resistant to activities involving touching.

(Thanks to Gina Dowding.)

8.15 ACTIVITY: snapshot

Aims

- To encourage women to be open about what they are feeling about the group.
- To encourage women to listen to what others are saying.

Materials

None.

Method **Time: 15–20 minutes**

1. Ask women to sit in circle.
2. Each woman to turn to the woman on her right and for five minutes describe how she feels about the group at that particular moment, including some analysis of what is going on in the group.
3. Change over.
4. Each woman feeds back to the whole group the information she has heard from her partner.

Possible outcomes

- This is also an exercise in perception and understanding: there will be gaps between what is felt, said, heard, and fed back. It can be very useful for women to watch this process at work in relation to their own contribution.
- When done throughout a longer event or course the activity takes 'snapshots' of the group, which become a record of growth.

(Adapted from WEA *Working towards change*.)

Mood lighteners/enliveners

8.16 ACTIVITY: fruitbowl

Aims

- To change the atmosphere and wake women up.

Materials

Circle of chairs.

Method **Time: 5–10 minutes**

1. Ask women to sit in circle.
2. Decide on four different fruits and give each woman the name of a fruit.
3. Ask women to repeat their fruit in turn.
4. Ask one woman to step into the middle of the circle. Remove her chair.

5. Ask the woman in the middle to call out one of the fruits. Those women stand up and run to another chair. The one who does not get a chair stays in the middle and calls out another fruit, and so on.

Possible outcomes

- Collisions, hilarity.
- Women with physical disabilities may find this activity difficult.
- Some women may find this kind of activity silly or a waste of time.

8.17 ACTIVITY: imaginary hats

Aims
- To ground women after working hard.

Materials
None.

Method **Time: 5–10 minutes**

1. Ask women to sit in circle.
2. Think of a hat they might wear that is real or outrageously imaginative.
3. Each woman describes her hat to the group.

Possible outcomes

- Laughter, amazement.
- Can also be used as an icebreaker.

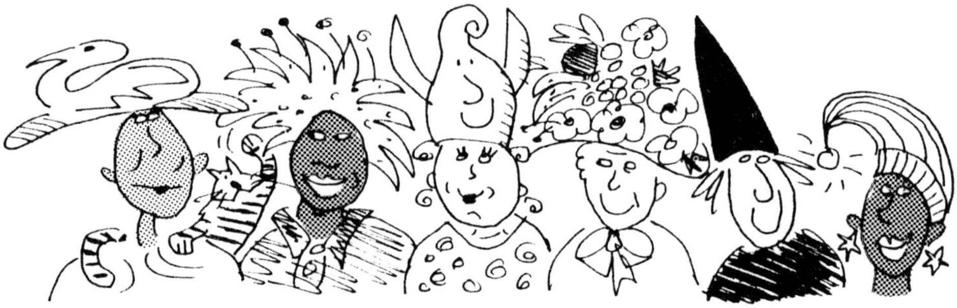

8.18 ACTIVITY: milling

Aims

- To change energy levels.
- To break up groups or cliques.
- To get group moving and facilitate contacts.

Materials

None.

Method **Time: 15 minutes**

1. Ask women to move around, trying not to touch and avoiding eye contact.
2. After one or two minutes, ask women to glance at other women they meet, but move on quickly.
3. After one or two minutes, ask women to meet other women's eyes and look at each other for two or three seconds and then move on.
4. Ask women to stay with the next person they look at.
5. One woman tells the other one good thing about herself.
6. Find another pair and make a group of four. Introduce each other.
7. Everyone could now be ready to start a new activity/session in groups of four.

Variations

- Evaluation: ask pairs to state one good and one bad thing about the day/event.
- Introductions: introduce women to each other by meeting and talking, then with another pair, and so on.

Possible outcomes

- Be aware that some women may want to sit this one out.

8.19 ACTIVITY: into a corner

Aims
- To liven women up through physical exercise.

Materials
Adequate space to move around, without chairs.

Method **Time: 5–10 minutes**

1. Ask women to stand in the middle of the room.
2. Point to a corner of the room. Ask all women to go into the corner who, for example, are wearing something yellow.
3. Point to another corner and repeat the instruction with, for example, 'all women who own a pet/read a newspaper/smoke', and so on.
4. Speed up as women get into the activity.
5. End with something positive that everyone will agree with, for example, 'Get into a corner all those who would like to see peace in the world.'

Possible outcomes

- It is no good choosing things that do not apply to the women present, or only to one woman.
- Women with a physical disability may have difficulty with this activity.

8.20 ACTIVITY: singing

Aims
- To use the voice as an enlivener.

Materials
None.

Method **Time: 5–10 minutes**

1. Ask the group to think of songs they all know (rounds are useful, e.g. 'Frère Jacques').

2. Sing a round either in small groups or pairs.
3. Ask the whole group to sing a song everyone knows.

Possible outcomes

- If the group is multi-racial/cultural it may not be so easy to find songs everyone knows.
- A popular song may be transformed by changing the words to be particularly relevant to the specific session.
- Be aware that some women may see it as a waste of time.

8.21 ACTIVITY: massage I

Aims
- To relieve muscle tension.
- To change the pace.

Materials
None.

Method **Time: 10 minutes**
Demonstrate the following to the group:

1. Shoulders: hand on opposite shoulder, roll the back muscle up and forward.
2. Neck: thumbs along edge of skull from ears towards spine; change to fingers and continue down spine; push the back neck muscles up towards head.

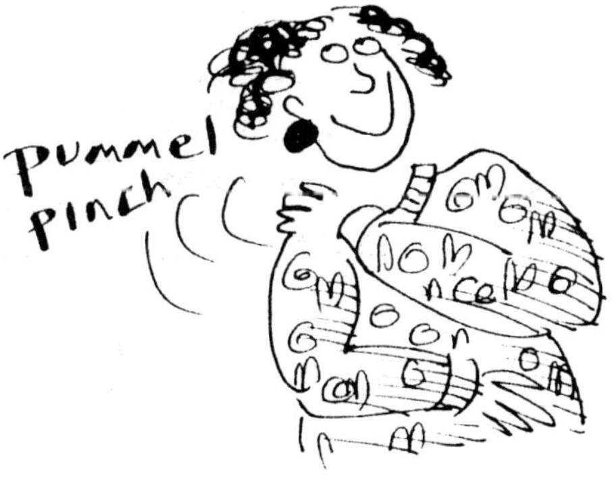

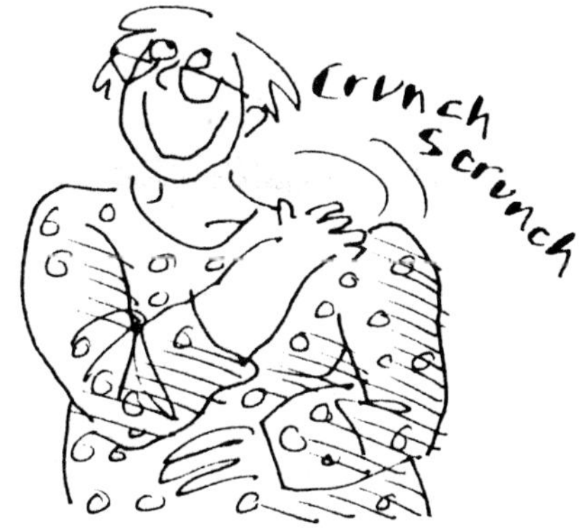

3. Forehead: start at centre of forehead, stroke rhythmically out and down to ears.
4. Eyes: close your eyes and place the palms of your hands, one over each eye socket. Let your fingers cross your forehead (darkness can be very restful).
5. Lips: with finger tips, massage lips over teeth.
6. Scalp: move scalp over skull with finger tips.

Possible outcomes

- Facilitator needs to try this activity beforehand.
- Women may be more receptive to self-massage than massaging each other.

(Adapted from *Women and health* activities and materials, WEA/HEC, 1986.)

8.22 ACTIVITY: massage II

Aims
- To change/lighten the atmosphere.
- To create group feeling.
- To make contact.

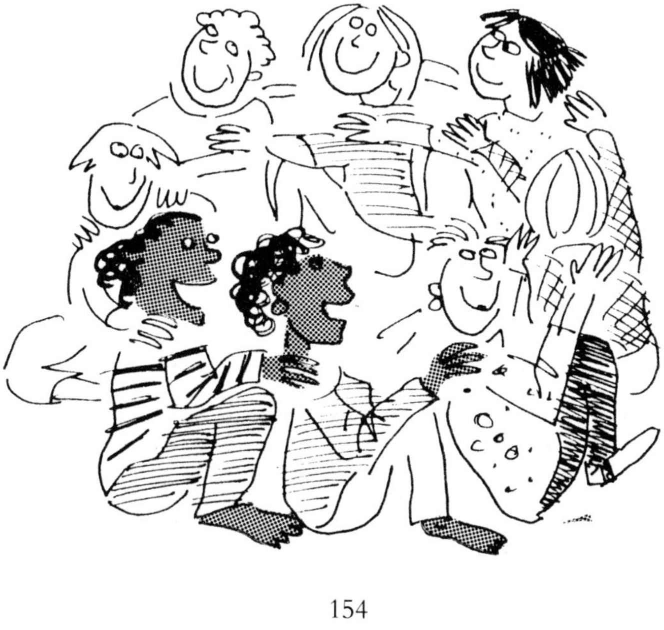

Materials
None.

Method **Time: 5 minutes**

1. Ask women to stand in a circle and turn to their right.
2. Place hands on the shoulders of the woman in front of them and give a light neck massage.
3. Stop when arms get tired.
4. Change places.

Possible outcomes

- Be aware that some women may not want to join in.
- Check to see whether anyone has neck problems before beginning.
- This can lead into more massage, and discussion about touching taboos.

8.23 ACTIVITY: relaxation technique

Aims
- To relieve tension.
- To take time out from 'head work'.

Materials
None.

Method **Time: 10 minutes**
Demonstrate the following to the group:

1. Stretch: raise one arm and reach upwards as far as you can. Let it relax and drop. Do the same with the other arm. Lift both arms, stretch, and let go.
2. Shake: shake arms loosely by side. Shake one then the other in a circular movement. Do same with legs.
3. Sway: feet apart, lean forward and sway a little. Let arms move freely.
4. Circling: circle shoulders backwards, first one and then the other.

5. Patting: pat yourself briskly all over – especially thighs and stomach.
6. Head roll: let head flop to left, roll across chest and up to right. Back to starting point, roll head slowly in a circle, then back again.
7. Hands: shake hands as if wet; clench and stretch several times.
8. Face: frown, relax. Raise eyebrows, relax. Frown and raise eyebrows together, relax. Smooth forehead with hands.

Possible outcomes

- Facilitator needs to have tried exercises beforehand.
- Women may feel easier doing relaxation exercises alone than with others.
- Some women may feel activity is a waste of time.

(Adapted from *Women and health* activities and materials, WEA/HEC, 1986.)

Evaluation

(See section 7.)

8.24 ACTIVITY: field of words

Aims

- To find out during an event how participants feel (especially useful on a one-day event, just before lunch).

Materials

Worksheet (page 157) for each woman.

Method **Time: 5 minutes**

1. Give a copy of the Worksheet to each woman.
2. Ask them to circle the words that come close to what they are feeling. If what they are feeling is not shown, ask them to write in new words, and circle.
3. Completed sheets are left in a pile as women go for break.
4. During the break, write up words circled on a flipchart, and record how many responses to each word.
5. When participants return from the break, they can see from the flipchart what the group as a whole is feeling.

(*continued on page 158*)

WORKSHEET: field of words

dissatisfied
reassured
positive
confident
helped
knowledgable
bored
challenged
confused
supported
uncertain
satisfied
tired
overwhelmed
indifferent
worried
negative
enthusiastic
angry
disappointed
tense
drained
happy
embarrassed
frustrated
out of my depth
relaxed

Adapted from "Greater Expectations" Szirom & Dyson, *Learning Development Aids* and taken from Health Education Foundation Course (1990) Stockport Health Promotion Unit.

Discussion points and issues raised

- Because this activity is anonymous, women are more likely to be honest about what they are feeling.
- If there are a lot of responses to 'confused', 'angry', 'disappointed', 'frustrated', and so on, then you will need to reappraise what you had planned for the rest of the event!
- If there are lots of positive words circled, but also words such as 'drained', 'tired', or 'overwhelmed', maybe you will need to slow the pace.

8.25 ACTIVITY: evaluation round

Aims

- To share feelings about the event.
- To give feedback to the tutor.

Materials

None.

Method **Time: 10–20 minutes**

1. Ask women to sit in circle.
2. If women's expectations were flipcharted at the beginning (see page 142), ask women to look at these again.
3. Women to comment briefly in turn on the event. Flipchart.
4. When finished, encourage women to talk about difficulties that have been voiced.

Possible outcomes

- Some women may have difficulty verbalising negative feelings.
- Some women may use the exercise to be critical of others.
- Include flipchart comments if typing up event to circulate to participants after the event.

8.26 ACTIVITY: evaluation guided fantasy

Aims
- To allow individuals to reflect privately on the event.

Materials
Comfortable chairs, prepared fantasy (see page 160).

Method **Time: 10 minutes**

1. Ask women to make themselves as comfortable as possible, either in chairs or lying on floor.
2. Close their eyes.
3. Tutor reads a prepared fantasy (specific to course/event).
4. After, allow time for women to sit and reflect.
5. Bring thoughts back to the present. When ready, stretch and open eyes.

8.27 ACTIVITY: evaluation in small groups

Aims
- To provide time for women to assess the event for themselves.
- To provide feedback for the tutor.
- To air feelings not voiced during activities.

Materials
Flipchart paper, pens, Blu-tack, Worksheet (page 161) or flipchart with questions.

Method **Time: 15–20 minutes**

1. Divide women into small groups with Worksheet or flipchart paper.
2. Give each group a set of questions, or put questions on flipchart. Read out and answer queries.
3. Ask groups to discuss and write responses anonymously on their Worksheet or flipchart paper.

(continued on page 162)

A8.26

Sample evaluation guided fantasy (will need adapting for your group)

Settle comfortably, close your eyes, and take a few long, deep breaths. Follow your breathing, letting your body relax. Each time you breathe out, relax a little more.

I want you to think back to the first time you heard about this course. How did you feel about it? Did you think it would be for you? Were you enthusiastic, a bit nervous or scared, keen, or was your arm twisted to persuade you to come along?

Move forward to the night before the course. What were you feeling then?

Think back to the first morning – the introductory meeting – coming to the youth club and waiting for the session to begin. Did you know people? How did it feel coming into the building and seeing other women arriving?

Then the introductions, and the time we spent making a course contract. Did you enjoy this? How did you feel at the end of the first meeting as you left to go home?

Think back over the whole course, and how you felt as time went on. Reflect on some of the activities we've done . . . looking at the roles and skills of tutors and group leaders . . . planning a first meeting . . . looking at different teaching methods . . . at discussion and role-play . . . issues relating to planning a course, and who decides – the tutor or the group.

How did you like the small-group work? Did you enjoy working with two or three others, pooling ideas? And what about the homework? Did you do it? Did you find it possible to make any time to do it during the week? What about the practical teaching plan? Did you find it interesting to be planning something on your own?

Now, the final session of the course. How do you feel now? How far do you think you've travelled during this course? Compare how you're feeling now to that first morning. What kinds of things do you think you've learned, and what areas do you want to find out more about? How do you feel about this group, and about the group leaders?

And the future. Where would you like to go next? Let your mind wander for a few minutes. Think about what use you hope to make of this course . . .

(Adapted from *Women learning together*, Salford Women's Education Forum, 1988.)

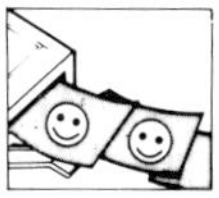

A8.27

WORKSHEET: evaluation in small groups

1. What have you gained from coming here?

2. Has it been what you expected?

3. Is there anything you feel should have been included?

4. Was there anything you felt uncomfortable or unhappy about. Why?

5. What do you think went particularly well today? Why?

4. Groups hand in their sheets.
5. Display sheets on the wall.

Possible outcomes

- Especially useful for large groups of 12 or more.
- May need to be followed with a closing activity (page 163) to avoid finishing on a disjointed note.
- If writing up event to distribute to participants, include summary of evaluation sheets.

8.28 ACTIVITY: Post-its

Aims
- To enable women to evaluate what they have got from the event.

Materials
Pad of large Post-its, pens, two flipchart sheets, Blu-tack.

Method **Time:10 minutes**

1. Give two Post-its to each woman.
2. Each woman to write something positive she has gained from the day on one, and something negative about the day on the other.
3. Put two flipchart sheets on the wall headed 'Positives' and 'Negatives'.
4. Women put their Post-its on the appropriate sheet.
5. Women read flipchart sheets.

Possible outcomes

- Women may feel more able to be honest because their comments are anonymous.
- If typing up event to be distributed afterwards, include flipchart sheets.

8.29 ACTIVITY: something I'm taking away with me

Aims

- To enable women to discuss what has been gained from the day.
- To give feedback to the tutor.

Materials

None.

Method **Time: 20 minutes**

1. Divide women into pairs or small groups.
2. Discuss together what they have learned from the event.
3. Back in large group, each woman in turn shares one thing she is taking away with her.

Possible outcomes

- Discussing in pairs or small groups rather than in a large group may make it easier for some women to be frank.
- Be prepared for negative feedback, for example, 'One thing I'm taking away with me is that it isn't safe to disclose private things . . .'
- Sample evaluation sheets (see pages 164–166).

Closing

★ 8.30 ACTIVITY: something I'm looking forward to/ going back to

Aims

- To ground women in the present and prepare them for leaving.

Materials

None.

(*continued on page 167*)

A8.29

Sample EVALUATION SHEET for a training day (to take away, complete, and return)

Please circle the number that comes closest to your views.

		not at all	a bit	quite a bit	very
a	Did you get what you wanted from the event? *Other comments:*	1	2	3	4
b	How useful did you find the event overall? *Other comments:*	1	2	3	4
c	How useful did you find the groupwork aspects? *Other comments:*	1	2	3	4
d	How helpful was it to share with women from a variety of backgrounds in women's health? *Other comments:*	1	2	3	4
e	How helpful did you find the event in terms of reviewing/developing your work or interest in women's health? *Other comments:*	1	2	3	4

(*continued*)

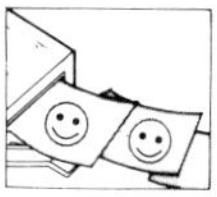

A8.29

(Sample evaluation sheet, continued)

f Can you suggest further training or support you may need to enable you to do women's health education?

g Did you find the crèche poor/satisfactory/good?

h What did you think of access to and comfort of the meeting rooms and the premises?

i Any other general comments?

THANK YOU FOR FILLING THIS IN!

Please return a.s.a.p. to

(Name and address)

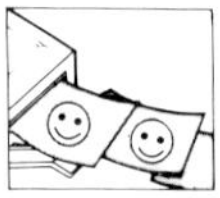

A8.29

Sample EVALUATION SHEET (open-ended questions)

Please complete the following sentences as honestly and completely as possible.

1. I thought the venue for today was . . .

2. Some of the most important things I learned were . . .

3. What I thought about the different teaching methods was . . .

4. Something I discovered about myself was . . .

5. The best bit for me was . . .

6. What I didn't like was . . .

7. Something I didn't expect to happen was . . .

8. I sometimes had difficulty with . . .

9. I'd like to use what I've learned to . . .

10. To do this I'd need more help with . . .

11. If there is a follow-up I think we should . . .

12. I'd like to add that . . .

Please return a.s.a.p. to

(Name and address)

(Adapted from *Women learning together*, Salford Women's Education Forum, 1988.)

Method **Time: 10 minutes**

1. Ask women to sit in circle.
2. Each woman in turn describes either something she is looking forward to or something she is going back to.

Possible outcomes

- Especially useful if event has been deep or emotional.
- Some women may not be able to say anything positive.
- There may be reluctance to leave.

8.31 ACTIVITY: what I can do

Aims
- To enable women to leave the event feeling confident in their ability.

Materials
None.

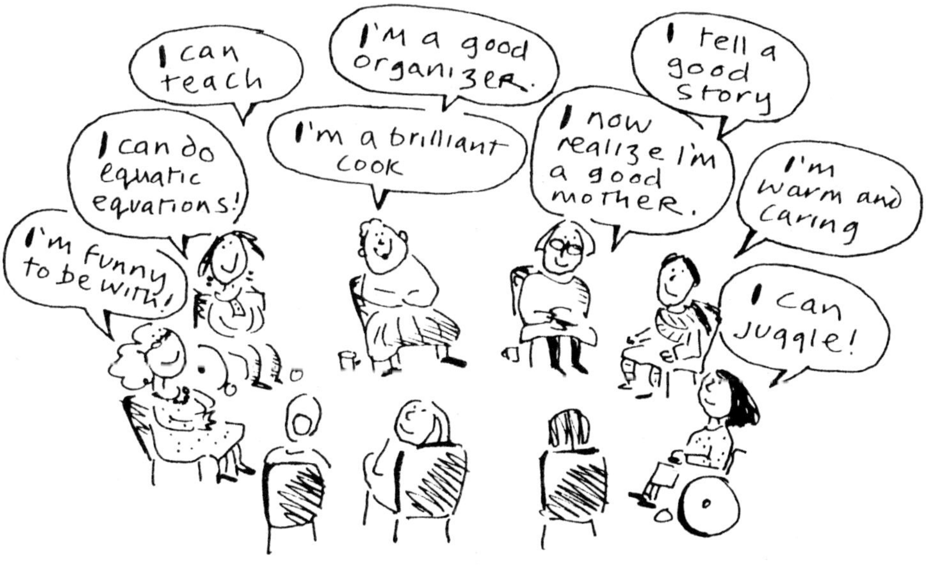
I can teach
I'm a good organizer.
I tell a good story
I can do equatic equations!
I'm a brilliant cook
I now realize I'm a good mother.
I'm warm and caring
I'm funny to be with!
I can juggle!

Method **Time: 5–10 minutes**

1. Ask women to sit in circle.
2. Each woman in turn identifies one relevant skill or ability she has, which she is willing to share with the group.

Possible outcomes

- You will need to have deduced whether the women will find it difficult to come up with a skill or ability.

(Adapted from *Working with uncertainty*, FPA Education Unit 1987.)

8.32 ACTIVITY: thunderstorm

Aims
- To end with a feeling of group cohesion.

Materials
None.

Method **Time: 10 minutes**

1. Ask women to stand in a circle.
2. Tutor stands in the middle.
3. Tell women to copy exactly what you do.
4. Look at first woman, rub your hands together.
5. Look at next woman, who in turn rubs her hands.
6. Continue until you are back to the first woman.
7. Move round the circle, clapping your hands as you look at each woman.
8. When you face the first woman again, start slapping your thighs. Continue round the circle as before.
9. Stamp your feet, and go round as before.

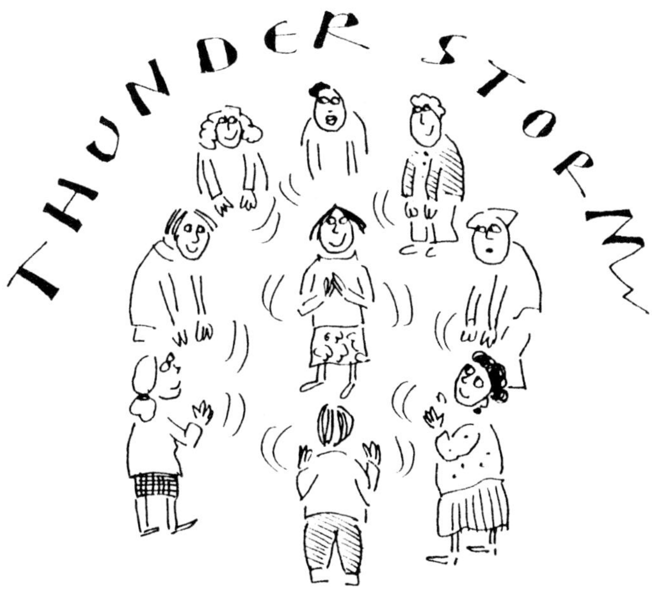

10. Working in reverse, move from stamping, to slapping, to clapping, to rubbing.
11. Face each woman with hands at your sides until whole group is quiet.
12. Thank everyone for coming.

Possible outcomes

- Especially useful if there has been discord or difficulties within the group.
- Be aware of women with physical disabilities.
- Some women may not show enthusiasm for this activity.

★ 8.33 ACTIVITY: positive strokes I

Aims
- To enable women to leave feeling appreciated.

Materials
None.

Method **Time: 5 minutes**

1. Ask women to spend one minute with each woman they have worked with during the event, offering positive comments. Stress that receiving a positive comment does not mean having to return one.

★ 8.34 ACTIVITY: positive strokes II

Aims

- To enable women to leave with positive knowledge of what others think.
- To have this in writing to refer to when confidence is low (a 'positive stroke bank'!).

Materials

Half-flipchart sheets, marker pens, and sellotape.

Method **Time: 20 minutes**

1. Fix half-flipchart sheet of paper to each woman's back.
2. Women write on each other's backs what they have liked about them during their time together. They do not have to write on everyone's back.
3. When finished, each woman removes the paper from her back, sits down and reads what others feel about her.
4. Take comments home to refer to when confidence is low.

Possible outcomes

- Only use this activity if you are sure everyone will receive a positive comment.
- Some women may find it difficult to accept that other women see them in such a positive light. Point out that no one was obliged to write anything, so comments are genuine.

(Adapted from *Sharing*, FPA Education Unit, 1987.)

Variation

- Put large envelopes clearly marked with each woman's name in centre of room.

- Give each woman small pieces of paper and ask her to think about someone she has enjoyed working with during the event. Point out that this activity is for telling women you value them, not for evaluating.
- Write down what she would like to say to the woman and place the comment in the appropriate envelope.
- When finished, distribute the envelopes.

Possible outcomes for variation

- Despite stressing that this activity is a positive one to show women how they have been appreciated, it could happen that women use the exercise to be critical of other women, perhaps because they had not felt able to speak openly to the women concerned. The facilitator should keep an eye on women's responses to reading content of their envelope.

Adapting a teaching method for different topics

Many teaching activities can be adapted to suit your own and the group's needs. The following are all adaptations of one teaching method: a game using small index cards.

8.35 ACTIVITY: contraception game

Aims

- To facilitate discussion.
- To help promote group interaction.
- To enable learning to take place between women.
- To liven women up!

Materials

Index cards with a different contraceptive method written on each, for example:

- pill
- sheath/condom
- IUD

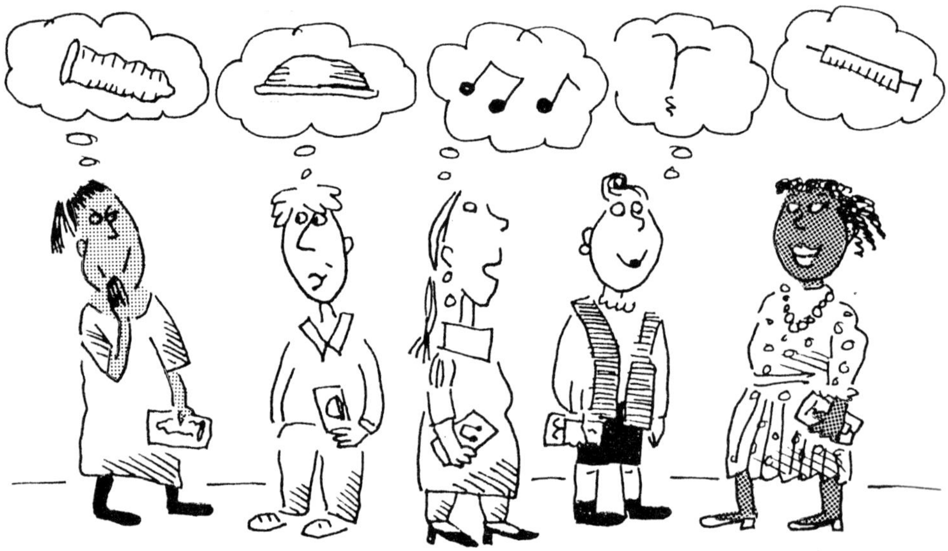

- cap
- injectables (Depo Provera)
- pill and sheath
- cap and spermicide
- no sex with men
- abortion.

Enough room for women to stand in one line.

Method **Time: 15–20 minutes**

1. Put cards in bag/bin/box and ask each woman to take one out.
2. Flipchart the question, 'What is the best contraceptive for women?'
3. Ask women to put themselves in a line depending on the method they hold, with the best contraceptive at one end and the worst at the other. (Allow 15 minutes.)
4. Ask each woman to read her card, starting from best along a spectrum to worst.

5. Discuss with whole group the issues raised, for example:
   - best in terms of least failure rate, or effect on women's bodies?
   - different levels of knowledge of methods;
   - contraceptive method as an individual choice, and so on.

Possible outcomes

- If women ask what you mean by 'best', tell them to decide among themselves.
- The line may start off in clumps of women. After 10 minutes you may have to prompt women to get in line.
- If lesbian women say this topic has no relevance for them, point out it may to the women they will be teaching.
- Some women may be unsure about the methods. Have back-up literature to hand out.
- Women may dispute whether some methods are in fact contraception.
- Can lead to a useful discussion about sexuality.

(Thanks to North Manchester Health Promotion Unit.)

★ 8.36 ACTIVITY: exploring dependencies/addictions game

Aims
- To encourage debate about addiction and dependency.
- To facilitate moving and talking within the group.
- To look at what is meant by women's health and women's well-being.

Materials

Small cards already written, pens.

- Ideas for small cards:
  - several pots of tea/coffee a day;
  - having a drink after work regularly;
  - smoking other people's cigarettes;
  - using heroin or other opiates;
  - eating chocolate every day;
  - using aspirin/paracetamol/ solpadeine often;

(*continued on page 174*)

- smoking 30 cigarettes a day;
- taking sleeping pills;
- using speed;
- sugar in tea with biscuits and cakes;
- taking prescribed tranquillisers;
- eating vitamins every day;
- jogging/aerobics every day;
- watching 'Neighbours' each day.

Method **Time: 30–40 minutes**

1. Give each woman a card.
2. Designate one end of the room as 'Sense of greatest well-being', and the other 'Sense of least well-being'.
3. Ask 'Which of the dependencies contributes the most to women's sense of well-being?'
4. Ask women to line up, depending on their card, ranging from best to worst. They can disagree, and move each other around.
5. When ready, each woman reads out her card, from least to greatest.
6. Join the group in a discussion, for example:
   - Why use 'well-being' and not 'health'? (Using 'health' can be too clinical, using 'well-being' can open up debate about what is women's health all about.)
   - Some dependencies are necessary to live in situations that are far from perfect.
   - When do feelings of well-being become detrimental to health?
   - What is the difference between acceptable and unacceptable dependencies? Does this make a difference to women's health?
   - How many women relate to two or three dependencies? Do they think they are dependent?
   - Is it silly to include chocolate bars and heroin in the same list? Why/why not?
   - What is the difference between dependency and addiction?
   - Why do you think women have dependencies? Are the reasons and types of dependencies different from men's?

Possible outcomes

- May bring up feelings for some women, which it is important to acknowledge, maybe ask how they are feeling, and offer to talk after the session.

- It may be necessary to split the group into threes and give a discussion point to each group. Allow time for discussion, then ask to report back in large group.
- You may want to cut discussion off at an earlier stage, as long as you mention some of the issues above in summing up.

★ 8.37 ACTIVITY: stress game

Aims

- To generate group interaction and dynamics.
- To get women talking and moving.
- To facilitate discussion about stress in women's lives.

Materials
Index cards, pens.

Method **Time: 30–40 minutes**

1. Give each woman a card.
2. Everyone writes a common response to stress for women on their card.
3. Collect the cards in a box/bin/bag.
4. Everyone takes a card.
5. Get in line ranging from most to least serious response, depending on card.
6. Each woman in turn reads out her card, from least to most serious.
7. Regroup, sit down, and lead into discussion, for example:
   - Are there clusters of similar responses, or are they all different?
   - What conclusions can be drawn?
   - Would a different group of women come up with different ones?

Possible outcomes

- Some women may feel the way they respond to stress has not been given the seriousness it deserves, which can lead to discussion about hierarchies and individual responses to stresses.
- There may be a need to look at what causes stress in the first place.

- It may be useful to get involved with the lining-up discussions if they become heated or bogged down.

Variation

Use small index cards already listing a variety of stresses (especially useful if women do not know each other and do not feel like sharing such personal experiences).

★ 8.38 ACTIVITY: safer-sex game: women and HIV/AIDS

Aims

- To discuss HIV/AIDS.
- To promote group interaction.
- To clarify relative risks of various sexual practices.

Materials

Index cards, each with a sexual activity written on it, for example:

- solo masturbation;
- vibrators;
- massage;
- french kissing;
- sex with fantasy;
- sex without penetration;
- oral sex between two women;
- mutual masturbation between two women;
- sex without touching;
- oral sex between man and woman;
- body-to-body rubbing;
- oral or vaginal sex between man and woman during menstruation;
- oral sex between man and woman with/without condom;
- mutual masturbation between man and woman.

Method **Time: 20–25 minutes**

1. Put cards in a bag/bin/box and ask each woman to take one.
2. Based on their card, line up from 'most risky' to 'least risky' sexual activity.

3. Each woman reads out her card.

4. Regroup and discuss.

Possible outcomes

- Do not assume women know how HIV can be transmitted.
- The activity can be threatening to women who do not know each other because it involves discussing intimate sexual activities.
- Some women may question whether some activities are sexual, which could lead to useful discussion about the difference between sexuality and sensuality.
- Women may raise the issue about how to get pregnant within a climate of safer-sex practices.

Activities for training others

- If women feel they do not have the skills to train others, they may need to validate the skills they have (see acknowledging and building on existing skills, page 178).
- There may be a lack of knowledge and understanding of how groups function, of group dynamics, and anxieties around problems in groups (see groupwork activities, page 184).
- Women may be unsure about how to plan sessions, how to approach the first session, how to deal with problems that might arise (see planning events, page 201).
- To integrate women's health education into their work, women may need to clarify where they would like to be going, what strengths and limitations they have, how to achieve what they would like to do, and to action-plan for the future (see clarifying/strategising activities, page 209).
- Issues around getting support and sharing with others will need to be considered (see networking, page 214, and support, page 222).

Acknowledging and building on existing skills

8.39 ACTIVITY: how others see me

Aims

- To enable women to get a clearer idea of their positive qualities.
- To enable women to value some of their own qualities not valued before.

Materials
Worksheet (page 179) for each woman, pens.

Method **Time: 15 minutes**

1. Give each woman a worksheet to complete.

Possible outcomes

- Women may be surprised by how many strengths others see in them.
- They may need help to see that their strengths are actually skills.
- Prompt women to transfer their skills to a women's health education setting.

8.40 ACTIVITY: validating and building on existing skills

Aims

- To enable women to be clearer about their own skills and talents.
- To help women to realise skills and talents they were previously unaware of.
- To value skills not valued before.

Materials
'Grid of skills and talents' (see pages 180–2) for each woman, pens and paper. (You may wish to simplify the grid in the light of your particular group.)

(*continued on page 183*)

A8.40

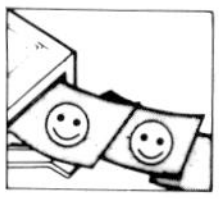

WORKSHEET: strengths and weaknesses

People	*Strengths*	*Weaknesses*

1. Under 'People', write down a list of people who know you.
2. Under 'Strengths', what strengths they see in you.
3. Under 'Weaknesses', what weaknesses they see in you.
4. Which strengths come up more than once?
5. Are there any weaknesses you regard as strengths, or vice versa?

(Adapted from *Getting started* WEA North of Scotland District.)

A8.40

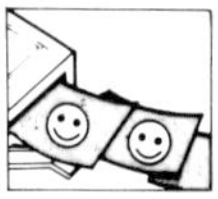

WORKSHEET: Grid of skills and talents

Skills	Recognised skills	Achievements 1	2	3
Skills with animals or plants				
Analysing				
Artistic				
Caring				
Communicating				
Co-ordinating				
Creativity				
Dealing with people				
Design				
Detail				
Diplomacy				
Efficiency				
Figures				
Food				
Hard work				
Healing				
Ideas				
Imagination				
Inventive				
Leading				
Listening				

(*continued*)

(Grid of skills and talents, continued)

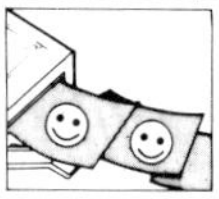

A8.40

	Recognised skills	Achievements		
		1	2	3
Management				
Good memory				
Money				
Organising				
Outdoors				
Patience				
Performing				
Persistence				
Planning				
Practical				
Promotion				
Relationships				
Reliable				
Repairing				
Researching				
Science				
Self-discipline				
Selling				
Solving problems				
Stamina				
Taking the initiative				
Talking				
Teamwork				

(continued)

(*Grid of skills and talents, continued*)

A8.40

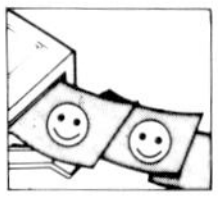

	Recognised skills	Achievements 1	2	3
Thorough				
Tolerance				
Understanding machines				
Words				
Working with your hands				
Writing				

(Adapted from *Getting started*, WEA North of Scotland District.)

Method **Time: 30 minutes**

1. Ask women to read through the grid.
2. In first column, ask women to tick the skills they think they have now.
3. Spend five minutes making a list of the main events or important things they have done in their lives, for example starting/leaving school, first job, getting married, having a baby.
4. Use the list as a reminder of things women
   - especially enjoyed doing;
   - felt especially satisfied with;
   - felt proud of.
5. Choose three achievements from this list that meant the most.
6. Using your new list, opposite each skill you think you were using, tick columns 1, 2 and 3.
7. At the end of the activity there will be ticks in three columns that were not in the column first gone through. The new skills can be counted up and compared with numbers of skills in the first column.

Possible outcomes

- Women may need prompting to think of things they have done that they feel positive about.
- Prompting also may be needed for women to realise the skills involved in their three achievements.
- At the end of the activity women will see ticks in colums 1, 2 and 3 which were not in the column they first went through. All the newly realised skills can be counted up and compared with numbers of the original ones.

8.41 ACTIVITY: acknowledging and building on existing skills

Aims

- To discover where skills come from.
- To validate existing skills.
- To examine what women perceive they need to implement women's health education in a group setting.

Materials
Flipchart paper, pens, Worksheet (page 185) for each woman.

Method **Time: 1½ hours**

1. Ask women to draw a 'map' of their lives in terms of events/people/experiences that have influenced/taught them in ways they see as important. (Encourage a few moments thought, downplay artistic talent.)
2. In small groups, go through Worksheet.
3. In large group, feedback and flipchart.
4. Lead into discussion on
   – value of formal education;
   – where and what do women learn;
   – is this a difficult activity to do? Why?

Possible outcomes

- If women have difficulties with drawing, they may prefer to work together on large paper to give each other ideas/support.
- This may need to be followed by a strategising activity such as 'Where do we go from here?' (page 214).

Groupwork

(See section 6.)

8.42 ACTIVITY: why groupwork?

Aims
- To acknowledge the benefits and drawbacks of groupwork.
- To enable women to be clearer about different ways of learning.

Materials
Flipchart, pens.

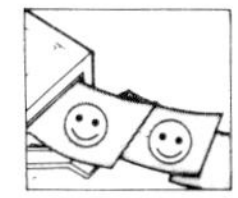

A8.41

WORKSHEET: Acknowledging and building on existing skills

1. What sort of experiences have been important for the group?

2. What skills and strengths have you identified?

Method **Time: 15 minutes**

1. Brainstorm positive and negative feelings about groupwork based on previous experiences. Flipchart responses.
2. Brainstorm what makes groupwork different from traditional ways of teaching/learning. Flipchart responses.

Possible outcomes

- Women who are confident about groupwork will contribute many positives; women who are new to groupwork may voice reservations.

(See working with groups in section 4 and section 6.)

8.43 ACTIVITY: roles in groups

Aims

- To enable women to learn about roles people play in groups by looking at their own experience.

Materials

Worksheet (pages 187–8) for each woman, pens.

Method **Time: 30 minutes**

1. Give each woman a Worksheet.
2. Divide women into pairs. Go through Worksheet and write down groups they belong to in everyday life, and the roles in each.
3. Back in large group, discuss.

Possible outcomes

- Women may express surprise at realising that they take on a different role depending on the group they are in.

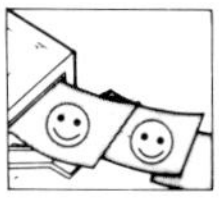

A8.43

WORKSHEET: roles in groups

In any group situation, people take on different roles, usually unconsciously, which help to strengthen the group. Below are some of these roles. Read them through, and add any others you can think of. Then answer the following questions.

1. Think of all the different groups you have belonged to and write these down:

2. What kinds of roles have you taken on in these groups? Use the ideas overleaf as a guide.

(*continued*)

(*Worksheet, continued*)

A8.43

Roles in groups

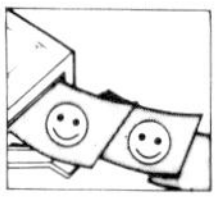

The initiator starts things off and gets the ball rolling. Often this will be the person who has brought together the group and who may be seen as the leader. It also includes those who change the direction of the group, bring in new ideas, and so on.

The clarifier tries to find out exactly what someone is saying, encouraging them to be specific and to avoid unclear generalisations. She also draws connections between what people are saying, and relates this to what the group is doing.

The information-giver offers to find information needed by the group, or has particular skills and experiences that will help the group.

The questioner will help the group to sort out what it is doing, and challenge assumptions the group may be making. She is able to step back from what is going on.

The summariser pulls things together and helps the group check what it has achieved. This can be done by giving a brief résumé of what has been said so far, or by taking notes and feeding this back to the group.

The supporter shows warmth to other people in the group, for example by supporting what they have said ('Yes, that's a good point'), or including others or what they have said earlier. This support can be verbal or non-verbal (nodding head, eye contact, smiling approval).

The joker brings light relief, humour and an opportunity to let off steam. This person allows the group the chance to enjoy itself and each other for a short time. This doesn't include destructive humour or ridiculing people.

The sharer makes a personal statement about general issues to the group, and so shares something of herself. This helps the group relate on a deeper, more intimate level.

The process observer comes forward when the group is stuck and says something like, 'I wonder if we need to look at why we're going around in circles.'

Remember that the roles we take on in groups are continually changing, and often we take on more than one role at a time.

(Adapted from A. Satow and M. Evans, *Working with groups*.)

8.44 ACTIVITY: goldfish bowl

Aims

- To observe what happens in a group discussion.

Materials

Chairs that can be arranged easily.

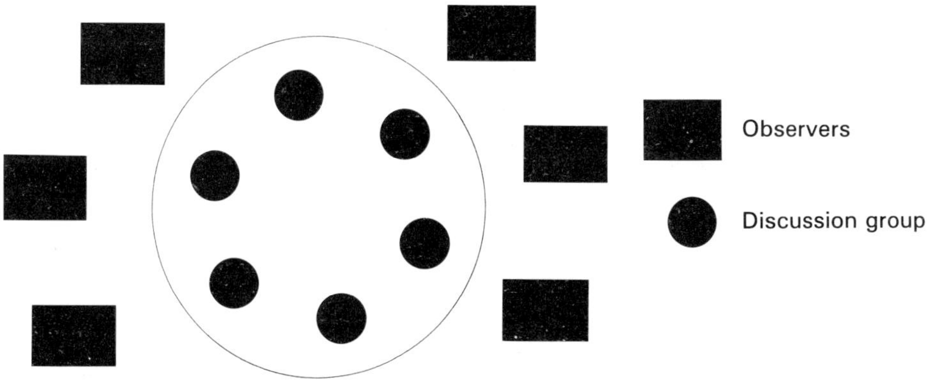

Method **Time: 40 minutes**

1. Divide group in half.
2. One group forms a small circle in which the women can talk easily to each other. The other group positions itself outside this circle so it can see and hear what happens.
3. While the inner group discuss a chosen topic as freely as possible, the outer group, the observers, remain silent. Controversial issues promote lively discussion, for example:
   – testing pregnant women for HIV;
   – embryo testing;
   – hormone replacement therapy (HRT) for older women.
4. After 5–10 minutes change places and roles, and choose a different topic.
5. Back in large group, discuss what happened, for example:
   - who spoke first? Why?
   - what roles did women take on?
   - who listened/responded most?
   - who did not speak at all?

- did anyone look uncomfortable?
- did anyone disrupt the discussion?
- how easy was it to observe without being able to participate?

(Adapted from Tim Bond, *Games for social and life skills*, 1988.)

8.45 ACTIVITY: what helps a group work well

Aims

- To separate planning, preparation, and groupwork skills.
- To formulate good practice for these.

Materials

Paper, flipchart, Blu-tack, pens.

Method **Time: 1½ hours**

1. Brainstorm:
   - What types of groups have women belonged to in the past?
   - What happens in groups that are working well/not working well? Flipchart responses on separate sheets.
2. In small groups, using the flipchart responses and personal experiences, prepare a checklist to ensure a satisfactory group meeting, using headings like: 'Before the meeting', 'First meeting', 'Group skills'.
3. In large group, report back and flipchart, and lead into discussion of role of facilitator/tutor.

Possible responses

Checklists

- Before the meeting
  - venue, access, publicity, targeting, directions, childcare, refreshments, handouts, own aims and objectives.
- The first meeting
  - welcome women, have a sign up, establish ground rules.
- Group skills
  - warm, encouraging, friendly, encourage equal participation, flexible approach, knowing what to do.

Possible outcomes

- Can lead to planning specific sessions.
- Can lead to looking at difficulties in groups that no amount of planning can insure against; the roles people adopt in a group situation, and some strategies for dealing with these.

8.46 ACTIVITY: role of the tutor

(See also role of the tutor, section 2; section 6.)

Aims
- To clarify the role of the tutor.

Materials
Worksheet (page 192) for each woman.

Method **Time: 30 minutes**

1. Divide into small groups and discuss the Worksheet.
2. Back in large group, discuss and flipchart responses.

Possible outcomes

- Because some women may be overawed by the number of skills needed, it may be necessary to move straight to an activity on validating women's existing skills.

8.47 ACTIVITY: feelings about tutoring/leading groups

Aims
- To clarify role of tutor/group leader.
- To gain confidence in individual styles of tutoring/facilitating.

Materials
Cartoon for each woman (see page 193), pens, paper, flipchart.

(continued on page 194)

A8.46

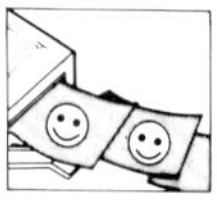

WORKSHEET: the role of the tutor

1. What are the things a tutor/facilitator should do?

2. What are the things a tutor/facilitator should not do?

3. What are the main skills a tutor/facilitator needs to have?

Common anxieties of new tutors

A8.47

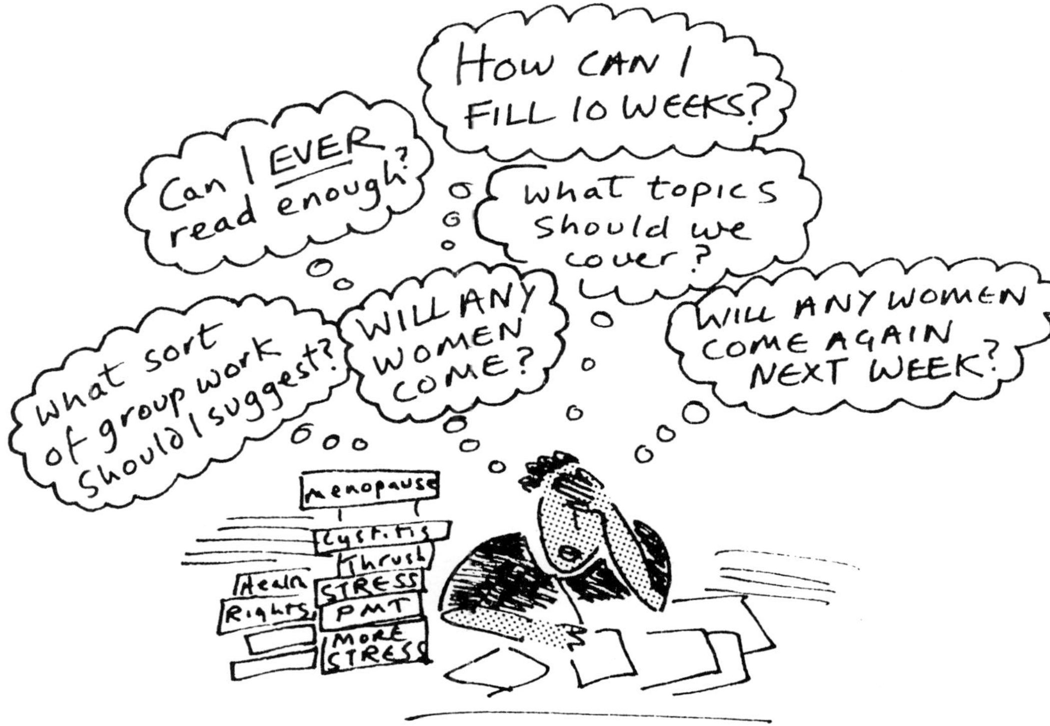
Can I EVER read enough?
How CAN I FILL 10 WEEKS?
What topics should we cover?
What sort of group work should I suggest?
WILL ANY WOMEN COME?
WILL ANY WOMEN COME AGAIN NEXT WEEK?
menopause
cystitis
Thrush
Health
Rights
STRESS
PMT
MORE STRESS

Method **Time: 1½ hours**

1. Give each woman a copy of the cartoon.
2. Ask if it reflects feelings around groupwork.
3. Brainstorm on anxieties about tutoring. Flipchart responses, grouping similar ones together, for example:
   - tutor as expert;
   - responsibility for others' feelings;
   - humour, personal styles;
   - disclosing things about self.
4. In small groups, divide responses for discussion.
5. Back in large group, feedback, flipchart responses.

Possible responses
Brainstorm might include:

- feeling inadequate;
- needing to answer every question;
- responsible for any feelings coming up;
- too humorous or serious?
- is there a right way?

Possible outcomes

- Does the traditional leader style affect perception about what tutors should be like?
- Does student-centred/participative learning demand a different tutor style?
- This may lead into looking at other roles in groups and tutor strategies for coping with them.

8.48 ACTIVITY: difficulties and roles in groups

Aims
- To identify different roles people take in groups.
- To look at ways of dealing with difficult group roles.

Materials
Flipchart, paper, pens, Blu-tack.

Method **Time: 1½ hours**

1. Brainstorm the roles people take in group situations (see page 188).
2. In small groups, discuss which you would find, or have found, the hardest to deal with. Why?
3. Feedback and flipchart responses.
4. In large group, look at ways the group tutor/facilitator could deal with them.
5. Lead into a discussion, adding additional ideas to the list flipcharted.

Possible outcomes

- Could lead into discussion of role of tutor and styles of tutoring.
- What roles are being played in *this* group? Encourage positive roles.
- If women use this to moan about groups they have been in, steer towards ways of dealing with such problems and taking responsibility to establish better working practice.

8.49 ACTIVITY: I could sabotage/disrupt this group by . . .

Aims
- To share problems that can arise in a group.
- To devise strategies to deal with such problems.

Materials
Flipchart, pens.

Materials **Time: 1 hour**

1. Brainstorm how women could disrupt the group. Flipchart responses.
2. In small groups, discuss how to deal with these.
3. Feedback to large group.

Possible responses

- hogging discussion;
- going off the topic;
- joking too much;
- abruptly leaving room;
- bursting into tears;
- yawning and acting bored;
- insisting on talking about own problems.

8.50 ACTIVITY: case-studies of problems in groups

Aims

- To give women the confidence to deal with difficulties in groups.

Materials

Worksheet (pages 197–200) for each woman.

Method **Time: 1½ hours**

1. From the Worksheet choose case-studies that are relevant to your group, or use the entire sheet.
2. Divide women into small groups, give each group the same number of case studies, but different ones reflecting a number of issues.
3. Each group looks at their case-studies (allow 10 minutes for each case-study).
4. In large group, encourage women to feed back case-study they had most difficulty with.
5. General discussion, flipchart responses.

Possible outcomes

- You may need to prompt women if they are struggling, and use the rest of the group as a resource.
- Try to ensure that small groups including Black women are not given case-studies dealing with racism.

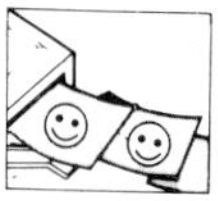

A8.50

WORKSHEET: case-studies of difficult situations in groups

1. You have put an enormous amount of work into preparing a session on common gynaecological problems. Half way through, you realise you are getting very little response from the group. Your attempts to elicit questions/discussion are met with silence.
   - What do you think is happening?
   - How can a group leader tackle such a situation?
2. Over the weeks you have become aware that there are two very talkative group members. They constantly spark each other off, and leave very little space for anyone else. You notice numbers are falling slightly, and that some group members are looking bored at times. You want to encourage everyone to participate equally.
   - What is the role of a group leader in a situation like this?
3. The group is mainly made up of young mothers in their late 'teens and early twenties. There is, however, a small group of 17-year-olds as well. They have expressed frustration at always talking about pregnancy and babies. They have also stopped attending regularly.
   - What can the group leader do to respond to this clash of interests/needs?
4. 'The women came expecting us to run the group for them. Many were acutely depressed and expected more assistance than we could give. We were out of our depth, our confidence collapsed, and the group folded.' (Health visitor and community workers – stress and relaxation group.)
   - What issues are raised here?
   - How could this situation be averted?
5. During a session on the menstrual cycle, one of the women in the group begins to go into a lot of detail about her irregular periods and looks to you for a diagnosis.
   - What are the limits of a group leader in such situations?
   - What could a group leader do in such a situation?

(continued)

6. You are having a general discussion about contraception, which moves on to first sexual experiences. The group atmosphere seems lighthearted and lively. Suddenly one of the women bursts into tears. You are taken aback and unprepared for this.
   - How could the group leader respond to this situation?
   - What issues does this highlight about working with groups and women's health topics?
   - What are the possible reasons for her outburst?

7. You are leading a women's health group. Today's topic is food. Suddenly, one of the women makes a remark about eating habits in other cultures. The remark seems to you to be very racist. You and the group members are all white women. You are taken aback by the remark, and angry. Your gut reaction is to tell the woman you will not tolerate such remarks, and to ask her to leave. Instead, you start talking about prejudice and imperialism. But other members of the group collude in the racism.
   - How could a group leader respond to this situation?
   - What issues does this raise about the significance of food?

8. Whenever the discussion turns to relationships or sex, Sally becomes withdrawn. One day the youth worker challenges her quite jovially: 'Come on, Sal, you must have some views on this!' Sally mumbles, 'I don't know.' She doesn't return. A few sessions later the youth worker asks if anyone has seen Sally. Two of her closer friends inform the youth worker that they no longer mix with her because she is 'queer'.
   - What can be learnt from the way the youth worker handled this session?
   - What kind of issue does this case point to?

9. You are a group leader running a session on food. The women are talking about their children's eating habits, and the problems they are having. You have two children yourself, so have experience of similar issues.
   - How can your own experience help/hinder?
   - Would you consider it appropriate to include your experience?

(*continued*)

10. You are running a stress and relaxation group. A Black woman is concerned about the stress she is experiencing because of racism. The other group members, though expressing sympathy, show no interest in pursuing this.
    - How would you deal with this?

11. The group is mainly made up of young mothers in the 20–30-age-range, with two older women. One of these in particular has expressed a need to find out more about the menopause, which she is experiencing at the moment. The other women have not shown any interest in this topic.
    - What could a group leader do in this situation?

12. You have been running a post-natal support group for five weeks, which has been well attended by a regular group of women. A Bengali woman with a six-week-old baby recently moved into the town. She speaks very little English, knows no one, and lives alone with her husband and baby.
    - Do you suggest she joins the group?
    - If she does join, how would you deal with the fact that she speaks very little English?
    - What response would you expect from the other group members to her joining?
    - Are there other support networks you could refer her to?

13. You are into your fourth session with a group and decide to prepare a discussion around motherhood, which involves dividing into smaller groups. The group is very resistant – one of the reasons they give is that it will divide the group and they enjoy listening to what the others have to say. You are particularly keen about introducing small group work as you feel some of the women are not getting the opportunity to express themselves, and the group is too large for an in depth discussion.
    - What would you do in this situation?
    - How do you work around the group's wishes on the one hand, and your desire to encourage women to try new approaches such as small groups or role play on the other?

(*continued*)

(*Worksheet, continued*) A8.50

14. You are having a general discussion about dealing with doctors and how difficult it can be to communicate with the medical profession. The entire group has been participating in a lively discussion. Suddenly, one of the women becomes very quiet, and then abruptly leaves the room.
    - How could the group leader respond to this situation?
    - What issues does this highlight about working with groups and women's health topics?
    - What might have prompted the woman's distress?

15. The group you are working with is looking at being assertive. You have carefully planned a role-play exericse for them, but the group is uneasy about using this method...

    You have a carefully prepared guided fantasy for women to evaluate during this last session of the entire course. Two women say they do not want to do it...

    One woman in your group consistently opts out whenever an activity involves writing or reading...
    - What might be the various reasons for the three incidents shown here?
    - What could you do?
    - What issues does this raise about choosing learning/teaching methods?

(Thanks to North Manchester health promotion team, for some case studies.)

Planning events

(See also sections 6 and 9.)

8.51 ACTIVITY: planning teaching sessions I

Aims
- To experience planning a women's health session.

Materials
Worksheets, A and B (pages 202 and 203), for each woman, pens.

Method **Time: 1–2 hours**

1. Decide which Worksheet is most appropriate for your group.
2. Hand out copies of Worksheet to each woman.
3. Individually, in pairs, or small groups, plan a session on a topic/issue.
4. In large group, feed back for comments/suggestions.

8.52 ACTIVITY: planning teaching sessions II

Aims
- To experience planning a women's health session.

Materials
Worksheet (page 204) for each woman, pens, flipchart.

Method **Time: 1 hour**

1. Give each woman a Worksheet.
2. In small groups, work through the Worksheet.
3. In large group, feed back and discuss.

(*continued on page 205*)

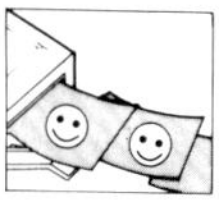 A8.51

WORKSHEET A: planning teaching sessions (2-hour session)

1. What is my target (number of women, their ages, specific groups)?

2. What topic/issue will I look at?

3. What methods will I use to pass on information and enable women to learn from others? (see section 2)

4. How will I add variety to the session?

5. Write up your plan:
   - aims
   - description of topic
   - methods and timings.

(Adapted from *Women learning together*, Salford Women's Health Forum, 1988.)

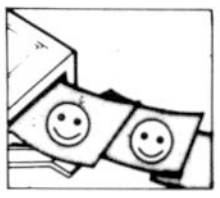

A8.51

WORKSHEET B: planning teaching sessions (useful for longer session)

1. What kind of group am I planning for (numbers, ages, specific groups)?

2. Will I work alone or with others?

3. How long is the session?

4. What are my aims and objectives?

5. What are the practicalities to consider?

6. How will I structure the session?
   - how will I present information?
   - what teaching methods will I use?
   - what resources will I have available?

7. How will I start/end the session?

8. What problems might arise during the session?

9. How will I evaluate the session?

10. Where will my support come from?

A8.52

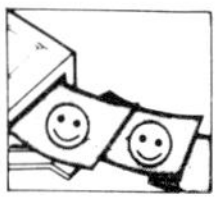

WORKSHEET: planning teaching sessions

It is the first meeting of a women's health group that you have been asked to help get off the ground. You have booked a local church hall and organised a crèche. You know of five or six women who have promised to come, but there have been many posters and leaflets, so you hope others will turn up. The meeting is to last two hours.

1. Before meeting:
   - what practical things need to be done and checked?

2. At the meeting:
   - what are your aims for the first meeting?

3. Make a plan of the meeting, to make sure you remember everything. List the kinds of things you would hope to cover, with rough timings. Try and agree in your group on a plan, and write this up on a flipchart.

4. What equipment will you need?

(Adapted from *Women learning together*, Salford Women's Health Forum, 1988.)

Possible outcomes

- A specific case-study to work with can be a useful focus for planning events.
- Small groups will come up with different ways of organising the same session, highlighting that there is no 'right' way.
- Large group discussion can point out issues not taken into consideration.

8.53 ACTIVITY: planning a course: who decides?

Aims
- To look at the balance between advance planning and responding to group needs.

Materials
Worksheet (page 206) for each woman and flipchart.

Method **Time: 30–40 minutes**

1. In small groups, study the Worksheet.
2. Discuss each statement. Decide what you like/do not like about each one.
3. In large group, feed back, flipchart responses.

8.54. ACTIVITY: planning for problems: the first meeting

Aims
- To look at the usefulness of forward planning to give women confidence.

Materials
Worksheet (page 207) for each woman and flipchart.

Method **Time: 45–60 minutes**

1. Hand out copies of the Worksheet.
2. In small groups, discuss each problem.
3. In large group, feed back and share strategies. Flipchart responses.

(*continued on page 208*)

A8.53

WORKSHEET: planning a course: who decides?

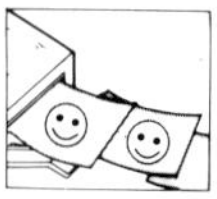

1. 'As tutor, I'm prepared to drop what I've planned to do if the group wants to do something else.'

2. 'I try to make the course content a joint responsibility between me and the group, right from the first week. In the end, though, the buck stops with me.'

3. 'My students feel happy enough with what I do each week, so I don't feel the need to change my overall plan.'

4. 'There'd be no point in my asking my group what they want to learn; they don't know as much as I do about the subject.'

5. 'How will I sort out what they want into a sensible pattern or structure? What if they suggest inappropriate topics, or things I know nothing about?'

6. 'I'll have to wait until I hear what they want before I can plan the course properly, even if that means thinking on my feet.'

7. 'There's no point building too much around what they want – I've got to get through my subject whatever they say.'

(Adapted from *Women learning together*, Salford Women's Health Forum, 1988.)

A8.54

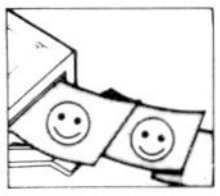

WORKSHEET: the first meeting

What would you do if:

1. Only two women turn up.

2. The door is locked when you get to the venue and women are already arriving.

3. You have just done lengthy introductions when three more women turn up.

4. On a one-day course two women come up to you at lunchtime and say they cannot stay for the afternoon.

5. A woman who has registered for your one-day course arrives at lunchtime.

6. The crèche room is next door, and the noise is distracting.

7. Your co-tutor phones just before the session to say she cannot make it.

8. Some women seem unwilling to talk.

9. The male caretaker keeps popping in.

Possible outcomes

- Feeding back into large group enables women to learn about more strategies for dealing with problems.
- Women may be pleasantly surprised at how capable they are in dealing with problems.

8.55 ACTIVITY: planning for problems: 'my greatest fear'

Aims

- To voice fears about running sessions.
- To share strategies for dealing with problems.

Materials

Index cards, pens, bin, flipchart.

Method **Time: 1½ hours**

1. Give each woman an index card.
2. Ask each woman to write down her greatest fear/anxiety about running a women's health session. Stress that what she writes will remain anonymous, though will be shared by the group.
3. Put cards in bin/box/bag.
4. Collect cards, shuffle, and ask each woman to take one other than her own.
5. Each woman reads out what is on the card she is holding. Flipchart.
6. Study flipchart:
   – Do some fears occur more than once?
   – Which are the most common ones?
7. Group similar fears/anxieties together.
8. Divide into small groups. Give each group a group of fears to discuss, and how to overcome them.
9. Feed back in large group.

Possible outcomes

- Women are more likely to state their fears because the activity is anonymous.
- Women may be surprised that others have fears similar to their own.
- Some women may come up with problems others did not think of.
- Sharing in the large group means women will learn a number of strategies for coping with a wide variety of problems.

Clarifying/strategising

8.56 ACTIVITY: stepping-stones

Aims

- To trace significant events that have led to involvement in women's health.
- To look at where women would like to be in future.

Materials

For each woman: five large white paper circles (dinner-plate size), one coloured paper circle, pens.

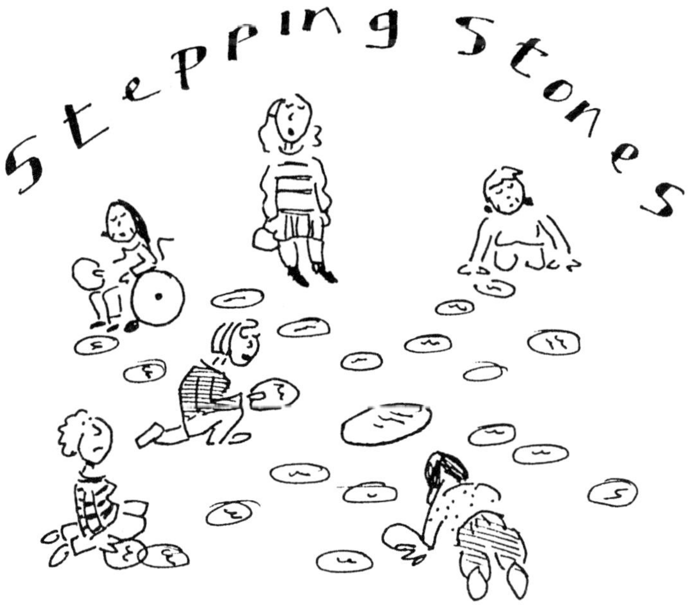

Method **Time: 45 minutes**

1. Give circles and pens to each woman.
2. Ask women to think of events/people that have been significant regarding their involvement in women's health education (they should only write what they are willing to share).
3. Write each on a white circle 'stone'. The last 'stone' represents where they are now.
4. On the coloured 'stone', write where they would like to move to next.
5. Place white 'stones' from edge of room towards the centre, ending with coloured 'stone'.
6. Walk around and look at 'stones', noting how similar/different the routes have been to women's health, and how different the first stone is to the present, and to the future.

Variation
To use this activity in relation to training, see page 29.

Possible outcomes

- Because this can be an intimate activity, with women sharing new, personal information, they may not want their 'stones' typed up with the rest of the event's proceedings.

8.57 ACTIVITY: SLOT exercise

Aims

- To enable women to clarify what skills they have.
- To look at how limitations can be overcome.

Materials
Worksheet (page 211) for each woman, pens, flipchart.

Method **Time: 1 hour**

1. Give each woman a copy of the Worksheet.
2. Individually, in pairs, or small groups, fill in the Worksheet.

(*continued on page 212*)

A8.57

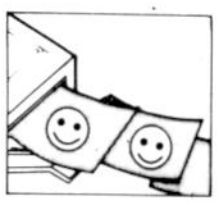

WORKSHEET: SLOT exercise

Think about your work in women's health education and fill in the following under the appropriate heading:

- What *strengths* enable me to do this kind of work?
- What are my *limitations*?
- What *opportunities* do I see for developing this kind of work?
- What might the *threats be*?

strengths	*limitations*
opportunities	***threats***

3. In large group, consider how to build on skills and opportunities, and how limitations and threats might be overcome. Feed back, flipchart responses.

Possible outcomes

- There may be overlaps between categories.
- If working individually, women may find it difficult to think of all the strengths they have.
- Women may well find it easier to begin with to fill in 'limitations' and 'threats', and may need prompting to see 'strengths' and 'opportunities'.
- Consider in large group how to build on opportunities. Discuss how threats might be overcome. Women may be able to share ideas here.

(Adapted from *Women and health activities and materials*, WEA/HEC, 1986.)

8.58 ACTIVITY: moving forward – action wheel

Aims

- To make a specific action-plan.

Materials

Worksheet (page 213) for each woman, pens.

Method **Time: 30 minutes**

1. Give each woman a Worksheet.
2. Working alone, in pairs or in small groups, work clockwise through the wheel, filling in each of the segments.
3. Try to determine what the first step will be.

Possible outcomes

- If women are working on 'action wheel' individually, they may find it difficult, in which case encourage women to work in twos or threes to help prompt each other.

A8.58

WORKSHEET: action wheel

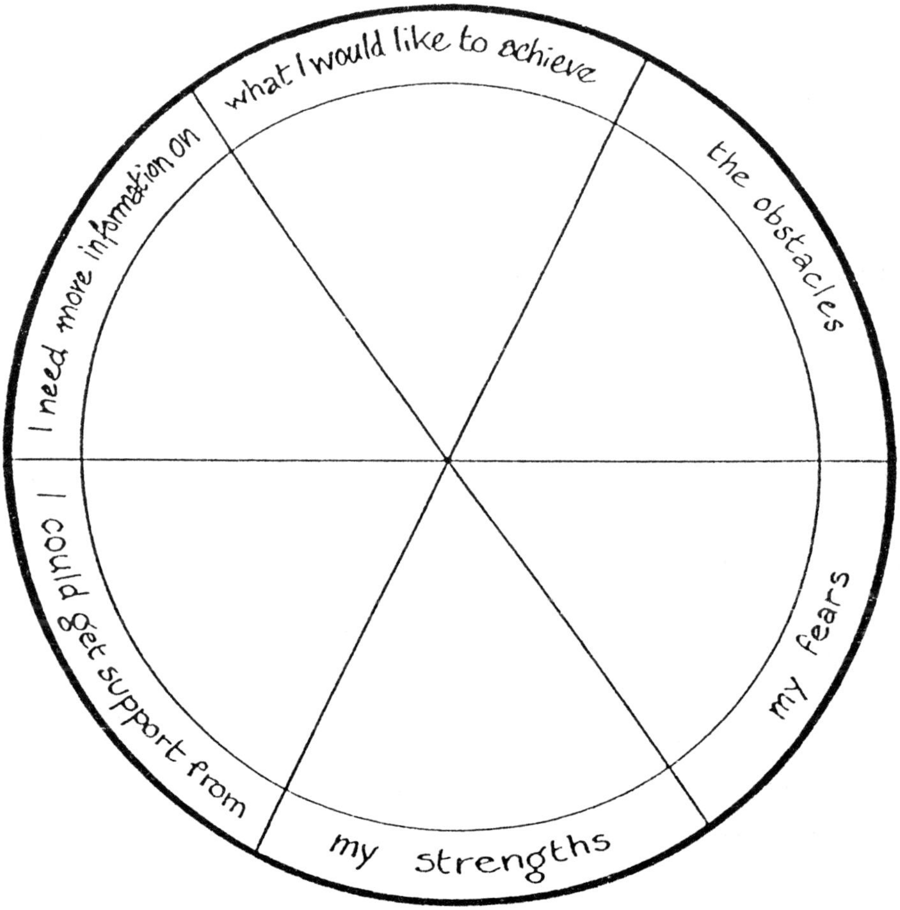

5. My first step will be ....

....

8.59 ACTIVITY: where to next? Sample action worksheets

Aims

- To identify next steps in women's health education and how to achieve them.

Materials

Worksheets A, B, and C (pages 215, 216 and 217) for each woman, pens.

Method **Time: 30 minutes–2 hours**

1. Decide which Worksheet is most appropriate for your group, or make your own.
2. Give each woman a copy of the Worksheet.
3. Individually or in pairs, work through the Worksheet.

Possible outcomes

- It may be helpful for women to share their action plans in the large group. Feeding back to the large group may mean more ideas for possible ways forward.
- Women working on their own might find it difficult to plan ahead. It may be easier in pairs or in small groups.
- If a follow-up session is planned, ask women to share what they have managed to achieve, and look especially at the difficulties they have experienced.

Networking

8.60 ACTIVITY: what is networking? I

Aims

- To clarify what networking means.
- To consider its usefulness.
- To encourage women to begin to network.

(*continued on page 218*)

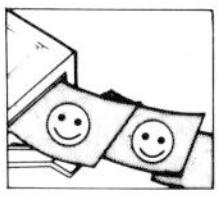 A8.59

ACTION WORKSHEET A (short course)

1. What possibilities are there for developing women's health courses in my area of work?

2. Do I foresee any difficulties/obstacles? How might they be overcome?

3. What support will I need?

4. What resources will I need? Where will these come from?

5. What kinds of further training am I interested in?

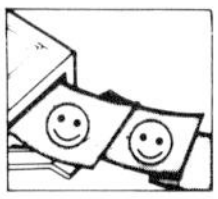

A8.59

ACTION WORKSHEET B (long course)

1. What is my goal? Is it:
   - specific?
   - measurable?
   - achievable?
   - realistic?
   - time-related?
   - worthwhile?

2. How will I achieve it?

3. What support will I need?

4. When will I achieve it?

5. What other barriers might there be?

6. What am I gaining by not doing it?

7. How will I celebrate when I have done it?

(From *Working with uncertainty*, FPA Education Unit/AIDS Education Unit.)

A8.59

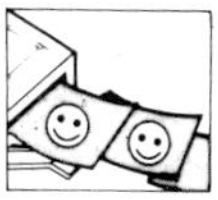

ACTION WORKSHEET C (short session)

1. What have I learned on this session/course that I can use in my own work?

2. What obstacles are there in me or in my work setting that might prevent me doing this?

3. How will I overcome these barriers?

4. What are my priorities?

5. How am I going to achieve them?

(From *Working with uncertainty*, FPA Education Unit/AIDS Education Unit.)

Materials
Worksheet (page 219) for each woman, flipchart.

Method **Time 30–60 minutes**

1. Brainstorm from Worksheet, flipchart responses or work in pairs/small groups and share in large group.

Possible responses (Brainstorm from multidisciplinary 'training trainers' event)

1. What is networking?
   - disseminating/pooling information;
   - telephone 'trees';
   - reaching out;
   - communicating;
   - working together;
   - linking people with common interests;
   - two-way traffic.
2. How do we network?
   - telephones/newsletters/mailings;
   - meetings/conferences/training events;
   - socialising;
   - word-of-mouth;
   - using the media;
   - campaigning;
   - lobbying.
3. What are the advantages of networking?
   - sharing/informing/supporting;
   - speed;
   - linking;
   - participating;
   - making contact;
   - pooling skills and resources;
   - increasing credibility/recognition;
   - exploring different ways of working;
   - power base;
   - avoiding duplication.

(*continued on page 220*)

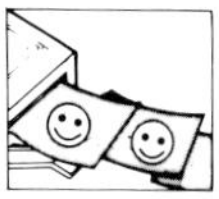

A8.60

WORKSHEET

What is networking?

How do we network?

Why network?

What are the advantages of networking?

What are the contradictions of networking?

4. What are the disadvantages of networking?
   – cannot keep up (time, lack of resources);
   – exclusion leading to alienation, cliques;
   – can become one-way/top-down process;
   – inefficiency/duplication;
   – lack of structure and aims.

Possible outcomes

- May encourage women to begin networking with others involved in the session, or wider.
- Women may feel able to strengthen an existing network.
- Women may realise the value of support.
- May need to point out that networks do not last forever; new forms with different priorities evolve.

8.61 ACTIVITY: what is networking? II

Aims

- To clarify what networking means.
- To identify women's networks.
- To find new networks.
- To discover ways of using networks and making them accessible.

Materials

Pens, paper, flipchart, Blu-tack, and Post-its.

Method **Time: 1½ hours**

1. Brainstorm what the word 'networking' means. Flipchart responses.
2. Each woman illustrates own network by putting self in the centre and drawing a 'web' of contacts.

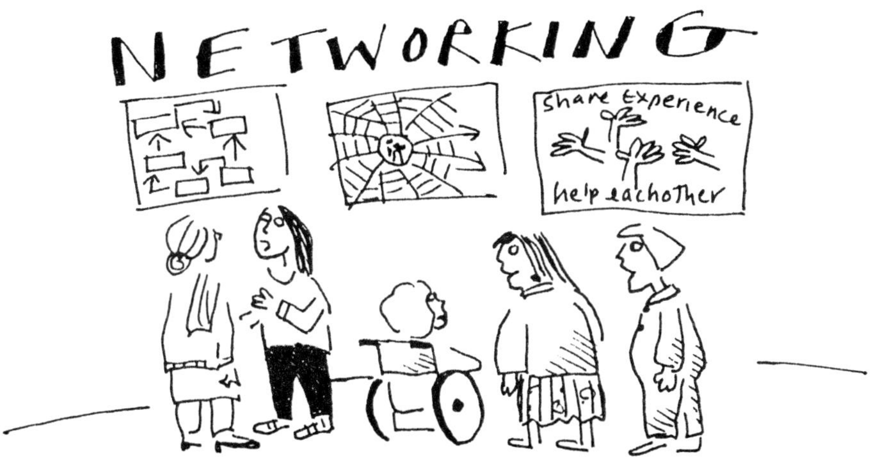

3. In small groups, share networks. Make a list of useful contacts, including group members. Feedback and flipchart.
4. Put flipcharts on wall. Ask women to put their names to contacts/groups using Post-its. After the session, type flipcharts and distribute.
5. Back in small groups, consider and list:
   – how to use the networks identified;
   – what is wanted from this network;
   – how to get what is wanted.
6. Back in large group, feed back and flipchart responses.

Possible outcomes

- Some women may feel they have little to offer and have difficulty drawing their own network. Facilitator might offer help and clarification.
- What women can get from networking is just as important as what they have to offer.
- If women feel they are lacking contacts, examine what they feel they need and where they might look.
- Consider local and national contacts, with a view to extending networks.

Support

8.62 ACTIVITY: my support group

Aims
- To discover individual support networks.

Materials
Worksheet (page 223) for each woman, pens.

Method **Time: 15–30 minutes**

1. Give each woman a Worksheet.
2. Work individually, in pairs, or in small groups, to complete the worksheet.

8.63 ACTIVITY: support, please!

Aims
- To clarify what types of support women need.
- To consider how these needs might be met.

Materials
Copy of Worksheet (page 224) for each woman, pens, flipchart.

Method **Time: 30 minutes**

1. Give each woman a copy of Worksheet. Fill in individually.
2. When ready, pair up to share or prompt each other.
3. In large group, flipchart responses.
4. Look at similarities in kinds of support.
5. Discuss where support might come from.

(*continued on page 225*)

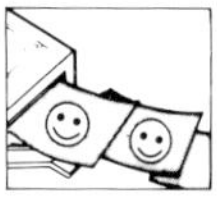

A8.62

WORKSHEET: my support group

Who do I know who will:	Friend	Colleague
Let me cry		
Listen and not get bored		
Give me a hug		
Always be honest		
Give me constructive criticism		
Let me be myself		
Laugh with me		
Celebrate with me		
Will not tell me it could have been worse		
Will not betray a confidence		
Will not say 'pull yourself together'		

(Thanks to Blackpool Well Women Centre for the idea.)

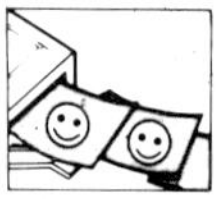

A8.63

WORKSHEET: support, please!

1. What kinds of support do I need in my work in women's health?

2. How might I get the support I need?

Possible responses
Possible kinds of support:

- Organisational
  - managers/colleagues
  - administrative
  - venue/crèche
  - other women to work with
  - forum for sounding ideas
  - validation of work
  - networking
- Resources
  - money
  - time
  - books
  - photocopying
  - handouts
  - video equipment
- Family/friends
  - understanding when you are stressed/overworked
  - act as sounding board
  - share your excitement

Links with other sections

This section can be linked with every other section of the handbook.

Resources

This resource section includes publications and organisations giving information on specific women's health topics, as well as resources on running health sessions.

See also: General resources section 11
for resources on differences between women see Resources, section 5

Books

Bond, T. *Games for social and life skills* (1988). Hutchinson, London. £8.95.
A collection of more than 80 games which teach a variety of skills.

Dixon, H. and Gordon, P. *Working with uncertainty: a handbook for those involved in training on HIV and AIDS* (1987). FPA Education Unit and AIDS Education Unit, Cambridge Health Authority.
(Superseded by *second edition* 1990 Family Planning Association). Available from FPA Bookshop, 27–35 Mortimer Street, London W1N 7RJ. Telephone: 071 436 3288. £12.99 + p.&p.

Ewles, Linda and Simnet, Ina. *Promoting health – a practical guide to health education* (1985). J. Wiley & Sons, London. £5.85.

Gingerbread/Community Education Development Centre. *Just me and the kids – a manual for lone parents* (1990). Bedford Square Press. £4.95.
Excellent resource, highlighting both the pleasures and problems of single parenting. The case histories could provide the basis for a discussion of mothering and health, and the book as a whole would be useful reading for groups intending to provide crèches, childcare, and so on.

Health Education Council. *Women and smoking: a handbook for action* (1986). Available from Health Education Authority, Hamilton House, Mabledon Place, London WC1H 9TX. £2.
A practical guide to activities for women taking action on smoking, many of which could be adapted or used as ideas for tackling other health issues.

Heather, B. *Sharing: a handbook for those involved in training in personal relationships and sexuality* second edition (1987). FPA Education Unit. Available from FPA Bookshop, 27–35 Mortimer Street, London, W1N 7RJ. Telephone: 071 436 3288. £9.99 + p.&p.

Kapit, Wynn and Elson, Lawrence. *The anatomy colouring book* (1977). Harper & Row, New York. Available from Green Farm Nutrition Centre, Burwash Common, East Sussex TN19 7LX. Telephone: 0435 882180. £8.95.
This book has large detailed anatomical pictures of every part of the body, which you can colour in and so improve your knowledge in a fun way. An excellent and popular resource.

Laws, Sophie. *Down there: an illustrated guide to self-examination* (1981). Onlywoman Press, London. Available from Women's Health (formerly WHRRIC), 52 Featherstone Street, London EC1Y 8RT. £1 plus postage.

Phillips, Angela and Rakusen, Jill, *Our bodies ourselves* (1989). Penguin, London. £12.99.
New edition of classic self-help reference book covering almost every aspect of women's

health and well-being with hundreds of references to useful literature, organisations and other resources.

Rural Unit. *Mental health in rural areas* (1990). Available from Rural Unit, NCVO, Regents Wharf, 8 All Saints Street, London N1 9RL. £1.50.

Salford Women's Education Forum *Women learning together: training materials and guidelines for tutors* (1988). Available from Salford Women's Education Forum, Education Office, Chapel Street, Salford M3 5LT. £2.00.
A course to develop skills in running women's education courses and groups.

Satow, A. and Evans, M. *Working with groups* (1983). Teachers Advisory Council for Alcohol and Drug Education and Health Education Council. Available from TACADE, 1 Hulme Place, The Crescent, Salford M5 4QA. Telephone: 061–745–8925. £16.50. Accompanying video available for free hire from Concord Video and Film Council, 201 Felixstowe Road, Ipswich, Suffolk. Telephone: 0473 715754.

Workers Educational Association (North of Scotland District) *Getting started* (undated). Available from WEA, 17 Victoria Park Squarte, Bethnal Green, London E2 9PB. Telephone: 081–983 1515. £4.95.
A basic education pack for tutors/organisers working with women in informal learning groups.

Packs

Cherry, Chris, Robertson, Marea and Meadows, Flora. *Personal and professional development for group leaders: a training course* (1990). Scottish Health Education Group. Available from Health Education Board for Scotland, Woodburn House, Canaan Lane, Edinburgh EH10 4SG. Telephone: 031 447 8044. £29.
This pack would be useful for women with experience of training and group leadership, who want to develop their skills. Based on training experiences in Scotland and Ireland.

Green, Felicity (ed.). *Health education foundation course* (1990). Available from Stockport Health Promotion Unit, 188 Buxton Road, Stockport. £25.
This covers the principles of health and adult education in a pack designed to be used over a period of six days. Useful activities, worksheets, and handouts.

Richardson, Carolyn. *Negotiating assertively* (1990). Available from Pavilion Publishing Ltd., Lansdowne Place, Hove, East Sussex BN3 1HH. £32.50.
This is a pack containing group exercises and handouts to develop assertiveness.

Women and health, activities and materials (1986). Health Education Council/WEA. Available from WEA North Western District, 4th Floor, Crawford House, Precinct Centre, Oxford Road, Manchester M13 9GH. Telephone: 061 273 7652. £6 plus p.&p.

Video/Film

Looking in the fridge for feelings U.K. (1981). Available from National Film School, Beaconsfield Studios, Station Road, Beaconsfield.
Thirty minute film on women and food presented by Suzie Orbach, author of *Fat is a Feminist Issue.*

Women and alcohol. Available from Alcohol Counselling Service, 34 Electric Lane, London SW9 8JT. Hire costs on application.
Thirty-five minute video dealing with issues around women and alcohol.

Organisations

Please enclose a stamped addressed envelope when writing to these organisations.

ASH UK, 5–11 Mortimer Street, London, W1N 7RH. Telephone: 071 637 9843. Wide range of leaflets on women and smoking, cost 12p each, send sae for publications list.

Brook Advisory Centre, Education and Publications Unit, 24 Albert Street, Birmingham B4 7UD. Telephone: 021 643 1554.
Write for current catalogue of the wide range of leaflets, and so on, which include contraception, sexuality, and sexually transmitted diseases.

Family Planning Association, 27–35 Mortimer Street, London, W1N 7RT. Telephone: 071 636 7866.
The FPA produces leaflets on all aspects of contraception, sexuality, fertility and AIDS. It also runs a bookshop and nationwide mail order service (at the same address).

GEMMA, BM Box 5700, London WC1N 3XX.
Support, information, and newsletter for disabled and able bodied lesbians. Newsletter available on tape, braille correspondence welcome.

London Black Women's Health Action Project, Bancroft Library, Bancroft Road, London E1 4BU.
Provides educational material for Black women on all aspects of health.

Maternity Alliance, 15 Britannia Street, London, WC1X 9JP. Telephone: 071 837 1265.
Leaflets on pregnancy at work, benefits for mothers and babies, teenage pregnancy and getting fit for pregnancy in eight languages, including Chinese, Bengali and Punjabi. Free to individuals.

National Youth Bureau, Information Services Team, 17–23 Albion Street, Leicester LE1 6GD.
Produces health information of special interest to young women.

Organisation for Sickle Cell Anaemia Research (OSCAR), Cambridge House, 109 Maves Road, Wood Green, London N22 6UR.
OSCAR have information leaflets on sickle cell.

Positively Women, 5 Sebastian Street, London EC1V 0HE.
Produces a range of leaflets around women, HIV, and AIDS.

Sickle Cell Society, 54 Station Road, Harlesden, London NW10 4UA. Telephone: 081 961 7795.
Leaflets and publications on sickle cell anaemia, including two videos (for hire), *Let's talk sickle* and *HB Master Sickle* (aimed at young children).

Women's Health (formerly WHRRIC), 52 Featherstone Street, London EC1Y 8RT.
Women's Health stocks a very wide selection of leaflets providing clear information on topics like menopause, hormone replacement therapy, HIV/AIDS, abnormal smears etc. Leaflets cost 30–40p each, plus sae, and some are available in various Asian languages.

Women's Nationwide Cancer Control Campaign (WNCCC), Suna House, 128–130 Curtain Road, London EC2A 3AR.
WNCCC has inexpensive leaflets on various aspects of women's cancers, including some in Asian languages.

SECTION NINE

Frameworks for women's health training

	What this section contains	**231**
	How this section can be of use	**231**
	Building frameworks	
9.1	ACTIVITY: planning women's health events	232
9.2	ACTIVITY: jigsaw framework	235
	Topic/issue-based frameworks	
	Two-hour session	239
	Half-day workshop	239
	Day workshop	240
	Ten-session weekly course	241
	Frameworks for training events	
	One-day events	
	Using the *Women and Health* pack I	242
	Using the *Women and Health* pack II	243
	Women's health and groupwork I	246
	Women's health and groupwork II	247
	Groupwork I	249
	Groupwork II	249
	Training issues	250
	Two-day workshop on women's health and groupwork	251
	Follow-up sessions	252
	Longer courses	
	Modular women's health tutor-training course I	253
	Modular women's health tutor-training course II	254
	Women's health tutor-training course	255
	Six-day course	256
	Problem-solving: when things go wrong	**257**

Links with other sections 259
Resources 259

What this section contains

This section looks at how to build frameworks for women's health events, whether they are topic/issue-based – for example, alternative medicine or older women's health – or method-based, for example, groupwork skills – or a combination of the two.

Previous sections in the handbook have given the *ingredients* for women's health events; in this section we consider the possible *recipes*.

- *Activities* to create frameworks for women's health events.
- *Samples* of frameworks for different types of training.
- *Ideas* for problem solving.

Differences between women mean that women coming to women's health events have a variety of needs, and therefore will get different things out of the same event.

How this section can be of use

- You may use this section for yourself by:
  - trying out sample frameworks;
  - creating your own frameworks;
  - appraising your own women's health training practice.
- You may use this section for training others by:
  - using the activities in 'building frameworks' in addition to activities around training (see sections 3 and 8).

Building frameworks

(See also sections 6 and 8.)

9.1 ACTIVITY: planning women's health events

Aims

- To consider the planning needs and possible outcomes of women's health events of varying lengths.

Materials

Worksheet (page 233) for each woman, pens, markers, and flipchart.

Method **Time: 1 hour**

1. Give each woman a Worksheet.
2. In small groups, discuss.
3. Back in the large group, flipchart responses.
4. Tease out planning needs that are:
   - common to all events;
   - particular to different-length events.

Possible responses

TWO-HOUR SESSION

- You may be going into an existing group where you do not know group members and they do not know you. Do women know each other? It is more difficult to pitch method and content for an unknown than for a known group.
- Are there existing ground rules? Need to make more?
- Topic-based/information-giving?
- Not enough time for the group to 'gel'.
- It's easy to run out of time.
- Need quick-and-easy evaluation method.

ONE-DAY EVENT

- Prior organisation
  - Crèche space and workers.

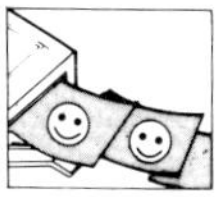

A9.1

WORKSHEET: what do you need to think about when planning

– a two-hour session

– a one-day event

– a two-day event

– a two-day residential event

– a course extending over a number of weeks

- Venue and refreshments (remember needs of women with disabilities, and special dietary and cultural needs).
- Pre-registration will enable you to find out approximate numbers of women, children, and what women want from the day.

- On the day
  - Can find out women's expectations about the day.
  - More time for introductions and ground rules.
  - Get to know women, women get to know each other.
  - Chance for more variety of learning and teaching methods.
  - Time to try different activities.
  - How to evaluate?
  - Closing activity?
  - Follow-up session(s) arranged?
  - Opportunity to network afterwards?

TWO-DAY EVENT

As for one-day event, plus:

- If the two days are not together, chance to give 'homework' in between.
- Can restructure or change format of second day in light of first-day evaluation.
- Women not turning up for second day?
- Will need different introduction/icebreaker activity on second day (see introduction/icebreaker activity in section 8).
- Check if ground rules are still okay. Need to add to them?
- On consecutive days women more likely to get exhausted! Need variation in learning/teaching methods and activities.
- Allow for spare time or women may feel guilty about opting out because of weariness.
- More scope for detailed evaluation.
- More opportunity for self-development.

RESIDENTIAL EVENT

As for two-day event, plus:

- May be more difficult for women to attend because of family commitments.

- More work can be done because women will be freed from responsibilities.
- Residential events are less likely to be close to home. How will women get to venue? Travel costs?
- Crèche facilities to cover evening activities?
- Informal, relaxing evening activities? (Some women choose not to have anything to do with alcohol, so may not want to participate in an activity based in a bar.)
- Emergency medical cover.
- May be harder for some women to leave an intensive residential event; think about closing activities (see closing activities in section 8).

COURSE EXTENDING OVER NUMBER OF WEEKS
As with one- and two-day events, plus:

- Get to know women very well.
- Attendance may be erratic.
- Group process more likely to occur.
- Lots of group dynamics!
- Scope for changing original programme, according to group's needs.
- Chance to use widest range of methods and activities.
- Where to next? Action plans?

9.2 ACTIVITY: jigsaw framework

Aims

- To enable women to share ideas for creating frameworks for specific women's health events.

Materials
Enough 8 × 5 in cards (or one-half pieces of A4 paper) for each woman, envelopes for each small group, flipchart sheets, markers, and glue.

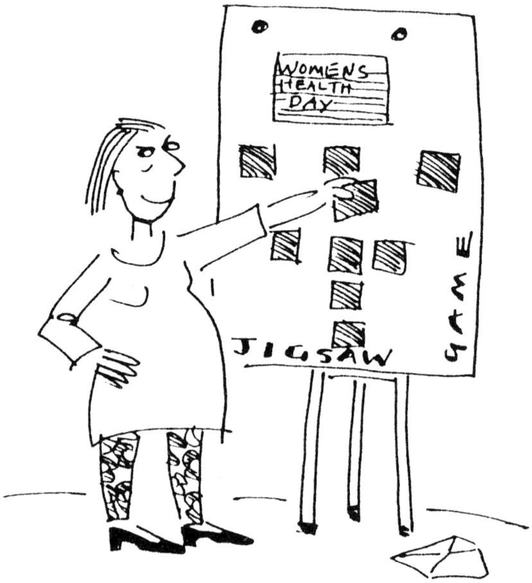

Each envelope contains four different-coloured pieces of card or paper on which have been written the following, one per colour:

1. Different process activities (for example introduction/icebreaker, trust, expectations, mood-lightener, evaluation, closing – see section 8).
2. Hostess suggestions (for example coffee-break, crèche, lunch, free time).
3. Training activities (for example acknowledging existing skills, groupwork skills, planning events, clarifying/action-planning, networking/support – see section 8).
4. Blank, for group to write down topics or issues.

Method **Time: 3 hours plus (see Discussion points)**

1. Ask each woman to think of a women's health event she would like to run that either is actually coming up, or is a fantasy; it can be topic/issue- or method-based, or a combination of both. Write down the details of the event on a card, with an eye to the prompts below.
2. Flipchart prompts:
   - How long is the event?
   - Aims of the event?

- Who is it aimed at?
- How many women?
- What age-range?
- Cultural mix?

3. Each woman leaves her 'event' card on chair. Everyone walks around the group and looks at all the cards. Each women selects one card for herself.
4. Form groups of four. Each group is given an envelope containing the cards relating to process and training activities/hostess suggestions/blanks outlined above, and flipchart paper.
5. Stick each event card on to the top of a flipchart sheet. Using the envelope cards, construct a framework for each event.
6. Afterwards, display all the frameworks around the room for women to look at during the next break.
7. The flipcharts can be written up, and the frameworks circulated after the event.

Possible choices of women's health events

- *Stress and relaxation*: two hours per week for six weeks; advertised to the public.
- *Women's health*: two-day multidisciplinary course for women working with women.
- *HIV/AIDS awareness*: two-hour session for Well-Women Centre volunteers.
- *Women's health day ('Taking control of our health'):* one-day event for women aged 20–70 from low-income, inner-city areas.
- *Menopause*: half-day event for practice nurses.
- *Assertiveness*: two-hour evening session for self-help group.
- *Hormone replacement therapy and early hysterectomies and ovariectomies*: one-day for practice nurses.
- *Women working with women in groups*: two-day multidisciplinary course.
- *Using the* Women and Health *pack*: one-day multidisciplinary event.
- One-day event for local women run by health promotion officer to look at *wider aspects of breast health.*

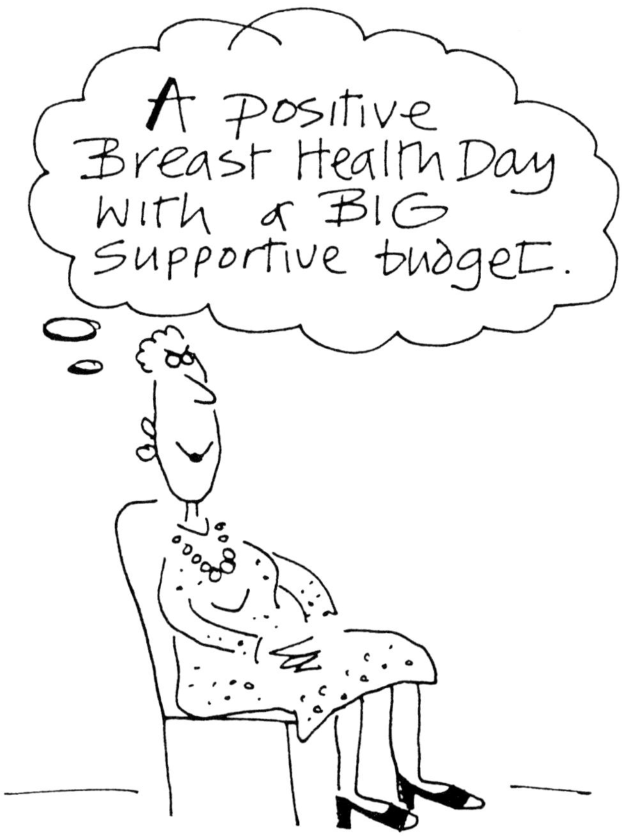

Discussion points and issues raised

- Time! Each event framework will take at least one half-hour to organise.
- Gives women the chance to share their experiences, balance ways of structuring a day, suggest new ideas, and help and learn from each other.
- Can be shortened by having four cards already written, each describing a different kind of event. Give each group one card to produce a framework.
- Writing up the flipchart frameworks creates a bank of material for a variety of training events, which can be referred to or used for ideas.

(Thanks to Sarah Clarkson for the idea.)

Topic/issue-based frameworks

(See also section 8 for examples of process activities)

Two-hour session

- Introductions if women do not know each other, icebreaker if they do (allow 10 minutes).
- Expectations – a quick 'round' will tell you whether what you have planned will suit (allow 10 minutes).
- Variety of teaching methods – depending on topic or issue, or to suit a particular group (allow 1½ hours).
- Evaluation (allow 10 minutes).
- Possibly information leaflets/handouts to back up the session, and where to get further information.

Discussion points and issues raised

- If this is a one-off session, there is less scope for altering the structure.
- If this is part of a course, there is scope for building on it.
  - Issues raised could be taken up in future sessions.
  - Could help leader and group define further training needs, and how they might be met.

Half-day workshop **Time: 3 hours.**

For 20 women who have pre-registered giving workshop preferences.

30 min	Refreshments and welcomes. Displays and information to look at. Children settled into crèche.
30 min	Introductions, icebreakers. Ground rules.
1½ hours	Choice of three workshops.
30 min	Short relaxation. Evaluation.

Day workshop **Time: 6½ hours.**

For 20 women who have pre-registered giving workshop preferences.

30 min	Refreshments and welcomes. Displays and information to look at. Children settled into crèche.
30 min	Introductions, icebreakers. Ground rules.
1½ hours	Workshops: topics/issues, choice of two (popular ones include 'Menopause', 'Dealing with your doctor', 'PMS', 'Dealing with children and staying sane!').
1 hour	Lunch (women bring food to share for an inexpensive buffet-style meal).
30 min	Getting back together. Game or enlivener, for example the 'Contraception game' (see page 171).
1½ hours	Choice of two workshops (e.g. 'Relaxation/massage', 'Looking at mental health', 'Assertiveness').
15 min	Tea break.
15 min	Group relaxation.
30 min	Evaluation. What next? Closing activity. End (relieve crèche workers promptly!).

Discussion points and issues raised

- These two frameworks are based on a session being 1½ hours, a fairly typical model in adult education.
- Women do not have to pre-register for workshops: time could be set aside during the morning to choose workshops, although tutors/leaders then must be prepared to adapt their material to the numbers.
- Selecting workshops on the morning of the event allows women to see how they feel on the day, and is not quite so formal.

- The minimum number of tutors needed is two, which can be increased to eight if each session is co-tutored by a different set of tutors. This can be useful for providing women with experience of tutoring with support.
- Crèche facilities should be offered at such events, and tutors need to ensure that the timing agreed with the crèche workers is adhered to.
- Leaflets or books can be available for women either to keep or to borrow from a library box.

Ten-session, weekly course, evening or daytime (with suggestions for possible topics)

Week

1. Introductions and expectations.
   Ground rules.
   Negotiating course content.
   Images of women in the media.
2. Dealing with stress.
   Listening skills.
3. Self- and body-image.
4. PMS and periods.
   Summary and evaluation of course so far.
5. Menopause.
6 Ageing.
7. Contraception.
8. Sexuality.
9. Breast/cervical cancer.
10. Evaluation and ways forward.

Discussion points and issued raised

- Each course and group will be different, and women will address issues in different ways, which might be related to race, culture, or class, and to limited access to resources.

- Working with specific groups of women will bias the course content towards group-related interests. For example, older women's groups may focus on ageing, osteoporosis, menopause and HRT, while Black women may want input on topics such as sickle-cell disease, or the effects of racism on health.
- One session can meet many needs: women may attend for information, or to extend their understanding of health issues – or to see how the course is run in relation to their own training needs.
- Some groups will need greater trust and understanding within the group than others, depending on the group. The group mentioned above waited until the final part of the course to look at sexuality and breast cancer; some groups may want to avoid such topics altogether.

Frameworks for training events

(*See section 8 for examples of process and training activities*)

One-day events

Using the *Women and Health* pack I — **Time: 6–7 hours**

Aims

- To look at ways of teaching women's health topics.
- To look at groupwork skills.
- To enable women to discover their training needs in women's health.

Suggested format

45 min Introductions.
Icebreakers.
Expectations.
Ground rules.
(See examples of process activities in section 8.)

If it is possible for the day's proceedings to be written up and circulated to women afterwards, tell the women at the beginning so

	they will participate more fully during the day, rather than writing notes.
2 hours	Using the *Women and Health* pack.
	• Look through the list of topics in the pack and choose one to discuss in more detail. Flipchart. (If only one woman has elected to do a particular topic, she will usually decide to join a group looking at another topic.)
	• Move into small groups per topic with Worksheet (page 248). Tell the women they will have 10–15 minutes to feed back to the large group.
	• Feed back to large group. The women will have gained detailed knowledge of one topic, and some idea of two, three or more topics.
	Lunch.
30 min	Getting back together again. Choose icebreaker or a game.
1½ to 2 hours	Groupwork skills. Choose activities on groupwork.
30 min	The way forward. Choose activities on clarifying/strategising.
15–30 min	Evaluation. Choose evaluation activity.
15–30 min	Closing activity (optional).

Using the *Women and Health* pack II **Time 6–7 hours**

Aims

- To look at ways of teaching women's health topics.
- To look at groupwork skills.
- To enable women to discover their training needs in women's health.

Suggested format

15 min	Settling the children into crèche. Leaflets and *Women and Health* packs to look through. Coffee and tea. Name labels.

30 min Introductions and expectations.
Timekeeping as group responsibility.
Ground rules.

15 min Introduce pack and organise first activity.
Choosing sections of the pack to look through – women choose specific sections of pack to look through in small groups and choose activity from within that section to try out with large group after lunch.

45 min Groups look at chosen sections using Worksheet (page 245). Choose and plan activity to do with group after lunch.

45 min Feedback in large group.

Lunch.

15 min Getting back again. Enlivener (see section 8).

2 hours Each small group tries out chosen and prepared activity on rest of large group (25 minutes per group with five-minute feedback after each one).

Tea during activity.

30 min Brainstorm: what are facilitation skills?
Discuss: what has been learnt today?
what else is needed?

15 min Summary of teaching methods used.
Evaluation.

Finish.

NB Women may need access to photocopier to reproduce worksheet from chosen activity.

WORKSHEET: using the *Women and Health* pack II.

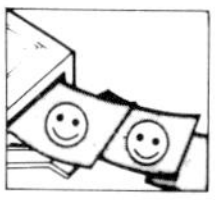

- What is useful in the section?

- How would you need to adapt material for specific groups?

- What activity will you do with large group after lunch?

- What will you need to organise for this?

Women's health and groupwork I **Time: 6 hours**

Aims

- To look at opportunities for developing groupwork and groupwork skills, and women's health networks.

Suggested format

30 min	Welcome/registrations. Introductions.
30 min	Aims. Hopes and fears. Ground rules.
30 min	Opportunities for developing women's health groups in your work setting (SLOT activity, page 210).
30 min	Coffee break.
15 min	Feedback from SLOT activity in large group.
30 min	Brainstorm: learning/teaching methods (discuss any that are unfamiliar). (See section 2).
1 hour	*Lunch.*
1½ hours	Difficult situations in groups. Either role-play examples of group relationships or look at case-studies of problems in groups (see page 196).
15 min	Tea break.
15 min	Local and national women's health networks. Brainstorm, or networking activity (see page 220).
30 min	Evaluation.
10 min	Closing activity.

Women's health and groupwork II **Time: 7 hours**

Aims

- To look at ways of teaching women's health topics.
- To look at groupwork skills.
- To understand how people learn.

Suggested format

30 min	Introductions, expectations. Ground rules.
30 min	Discuss what kinds of groups women work with or would like to and why. Flipchart responses.
15 min	Coffee break.
2 hours	Activity: learning from experience; how people learn (see Activity: learning in groups, page 84).
1 hour	*Lunch.*
30 min	Getting back together. 'Contraception game' (see page 171).
2 hours	Using the *Women and Health* pack • Ask women to go through a list of topics in the pack and decide which they would prefer to look through in more detail. If only one woman wants to do a topic, she will usually join another group. (Allow 15 minutes.) • Move into small groups with Worksheet (page 248). (Allow 45 minutes.) • Feed back to large group. Flipchart responses (Allow 1 hour.)
15 min	Brainstorm: facilitation skills. Flipchart responses.
15 min	Closing activity (see section 8).

WORKSHEET: using the *Women and Health* pack I.

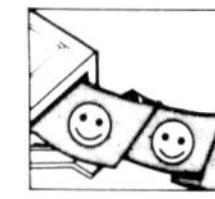

- What is useful about this section?

- Would you need to adapt anything for a particular group?

- What would you like to try out?

Groupwork I **Time: 6–7 hours**

Aims

- To look at what groupwork skills are needed for women's health education.

Suggested format

15 min	Children into crèche. Refreshments.
30 min	Introduction, expectations. Ground rules.
2 hours	Activity: what helps a group work well? (page 190).
1 hour	Lunch.
15 min	Getting back together. Icebreaker or enlivener.
1 hour	Activity: difficulties and roles in groups (page 194).
15 min	Break.
1 hour	Activity: role of the tutor; feelings about tutoring (page 191).
45 min	Summary. Clarifying/strategising activity (see section 8). Evaluation.

Groupwork II **Time: 6–7 hours**

Choose activities from section 8 demonstrating a variety of teaching methods.

- Introductions, expectations, ground rules
- Activity: why groupwork? (page 184).
- Activity: individual roles in groups (page 186).
- Activity: role of the tutor (page 191).

Lunch.

- Getting back together: icebreaker (page 137).
- Activity: my greatest fear (page 208).
- Case-studies of problems in groups (page 196).
- Where next? Clarifying/strategising activity (see section 8).
- Evaluation.

Training issues **Time: 6–7 hours**

Aims

- To look at networking and support as part of training.
- To elicit good practice for training.
- To look at blocks to achieve this.

Suggested format

45 min	Refreshments. Introductions, expectations. Ground rules.
30 min	Activity: checklists for good training practice (page 31). (Continue after break.)
10 min	Coffee break.
30 min	Continue activity. Feedback and discussion.
30 min	Activity: back to life, back to reality (page 265). Personal/organisational limitations.
1 hour	*Lunch.*
10 mins	Getting back together. Group neck massage (page 154).
1 hour	Activity: education and training (page 20).
15 min	Tea break.
15 min	Networking as part of training. Activity: what is networking? (page 214).
30 min	Support as part of training. Activity: support please! (page 222).
20 mins	Discussion: generating a model of training for women's health education.
10 mins	Evaluation with prompt questions using Post-its (page 162). • What have you found useful today? • What further training do you need? • Comments on organisation/structure. • What will you now go away and do? Finish.

Two-day workshop on women's health and groupwork

This combines the events on pages 242 and 249 to create a balanced, two-day workshop.

Aims

- To use the *Women and Health* pack as a training tool.
- To develop groupwork skills.

This event can be run as two consecutive days or with a break between. If run consecutively, it can be more intense and women will get to know each other better. Having space between the two days allows for tasks/homework and can give tutors time to plan the second day in response to the first.

When days are spaced out, more time will be needed for women to get to know each other again. Some women may not attend the second day as enthusiasm wanes or work priorities change.

Day one

- Introductions, expectations.
- Ground rules.
- Activity: using the *Women and Health* pack (page 243).
- *Lunch.*
- Feedback from groups/presentations.
- What went well/what could be better.
- Brainstorm: what are facilitation skills?
- Summary of teaching methods used.
- Evaluation.

Day two

- Names refresher, icebreaker.
- Activity: what helps a group work well? (page 190).
- Lunch.

(*continued on page 252*)

- Activity: difficulties and roles in groups (page 194).
- Break.
- Activity: role of the tutor (page 191).
- Summary of the two days.
- Activity: way forward (page 214).
- Evaluation.

Follow-up sessions

- These types of workshops usually will be a 'taster' for women.
- If already confident in teaching women's health using groupwork methods, some women find them sufficient for their needs, reaffirming what they are doing as well as giving them ideas and putting them in touch with women doing similar work.
- Other women find such events help to clarify their further training needs.
- Women already experienced in groupwork, such as community workers and community education workers, may feel they need further training in women's health topics or issues.
- Women health workers not used to working with groups may feel they need further training in groupwork skills.

Possibilities for following up one-day workshops

- A two-hour meeting one month later to work out further training needs, which are sometimes clearer after the event.
- Two-hour sessions every two months to meet and talk about work, as well as to discuss an agreed topic or issue. (Note: this can result in the group becoming introspective, without an agreed structure. If follow-up meetings are open-ended, the training process itself is never-ending.)
- A course of six, eight, or 10 two-hour sessions to look at groupwork skills or women's health topics or issues.
- A one-day workshop to look at groupwork skills.
- A one-day workshop to look at women's health topics or issues in depth.

- A course or workshop to include a combination of both women's health topics or issues and groupwork skills.

Advantages of follow-up sessions

- Will be responding to specific training needs.
- Participant-led training in terms of agenda and time-scale.
- Women participate who may not otherwise commit themselves to a fixed course on training issues. This may be because of limited time and energy, lack of confidence, not knowing exactly what they want until they begin the process.

Disadvantages of follow-up sessions

- If group needs are too varied, sessions may be lacking structure.
- Trying to meet all the group's needs and in practice meeting none.
- Limitations within a working environment where time for training is limited; approval, cover for absence, funding may have to be arranged in advance.

Longer courses

Modular women's health tutor-training course I

Components for each module:

Module 1 (two-hour, weekly sessions for 10 weeks.)

- First session, agree programme.
- Variety of teaching methods.
- Using women's health topics as training tool.
- Activities on groupwork skills.
- Ways of evaluating.
- How to plan women's health sessions: programme, publicity.
- Preparation for Module 2.

Module 2 Running actual women's health topic-based sessions (one or more two-hour sessions).

- Preferably working in pairs to support each other.
- Within own work setting.
- Setting up specific short course for women in the community.
- Recording/evaluating each session.
- Networking.

Module 3 (two-hour, weekly sessions for five weeks)

- Sharing experiences of running women's health sessions.
- As a group, looking at issues that came up
  - building on positive ones;
  - dealing with difficulties.
- Reviewing further training needs.
- Action-planning for the future – where next?

Modular women's health tutor-training course II

Module 1 (half-day meeting)

- Determining needs, expectations.
- Clarifying aims.
- Working together to construct a programme.
- Enabling women to get to know one another.

Module 2 (two consecutive-day workshops)

- Variety of teaching methods.
- Women's health topics as training tool.
- Activities on groupwork skills.
- Ways of evaluating.

- How to plan a women's health session: programme, publicity.

Homework: preparing a practical session plan.

Four-week gap

Module 3 (one-day workshop)

- Sharing practical session plans.
- Modifying session plans in light of comments/suggestions from group.
- Preparing for putting session plan into action.

Module 4 (extending over three-month period)

- Running actual women's health topic-based sessions (one or more two-hour sessions).
- Working within actual work settings.
- Recording/evaluating each session.
- Networking.

Module 5 (one-day workshop)

- Sharing experiences of running actual sessions.
- As a group, looking at issues that came up
  - building on positive ones;
  - dealing with difficulties.
- Reviewing further training needs and how they might be met.
- Action-planning for the future: where next?

Women's health tutor-training course (one half-day weekly, over 10 weeks)

Aims

- To provide the opportunity to learn about and practise skills essential to tutoring women's health groups.
- To enable women to reflect on and plan further development.

Week

1. Welcome, introductions, aims, ground rules.
   Why women's health education? (see section 4).
   Negative and positive learning.
2. Characteristics of adult learning (see sections 3 and 6).
   Principles of learning.
   Communication skills.
3. Group processes and roles in groups (see sections 6 and 8).
   Difficult situations in groups.
4. Aims/scheme of work/lesson-planning.
   Review of the course so far.
5. Learning/teaching methods (see section 2).
6. Specific health topics/issues.
   Practising learning methods – having a go.
7. Revising scheme of work.
   Planning groups or courses (see section 9).
   Preparation for micro-teaching – planning specific teaching session to try out on rest of group (see section 3).
8. Resources, equipment, books, contacts, networks.
   Tutorials.
9. Micro-teaching – trying out teaching session on rest of group.
10. The way forward.
    Evaluation.
    Personal asessment.

Six-day course

Day

1. Introductions, expectations.
   Agenda-setting.
   Using the *Women and Health* pack (page 243).
2. Acknowledging/building on existing skills (page 178).
   Groupwork activities (see section 8).
3. Planning and structuring a women's health event.

Homework: planning workshops/research.

4. Practice workshops/constructive criticism (micro-teaching).
5. Women's health event.
6. Feedback/evaluation of women's health event.
   The way forward.
   Networking and support activities.
   Evaluation of course.
   } (see section 8)

Discussion points and issues raised

- The women's health event can either be one single event that the group puts on, or separate events within different work settings.
- The time-scale can either be one day a month for six months, or a two-month gap between days three and four to organise the event in time for publicity to go out.
- The women's health event can be co-tutored, and can then be planned and researched jointly during the homework period.

Problem-solving: when things go wrong

- *Far fewer women turn up than you expected*
  This can seem like a disaster! You may not be able to split into small groups as intended, so try pairs instead. You may need to re-negotiate the programme. It may turn out to be a different event as a result – but still very positive!
- *Your programme does not match the women's needs*
  If the women pre-registered, you should have some idea of what they want from the session. Even so, it is useful to check their expectations at the beginning.

  If you have organised an event to which women just turn up, it is even more important to find out expectations and fears. If your publicity has been adequate you should not be too far off the mark, but sometimes women will attend with expectations that cannot possibly be met. Be honest at the start if this is the case; you might be able to suggest how their needs could be met.

  Sometimes women have a hidden agenda in which they want to do things differently from what they originally said. They will need to be referred back to their stated expectations.

- *You have forgotten to bring materials you need*
  We all do this at some point! Forward planning (see section 6) can keep this to a minimum, but even with the best preparation you can find yourself stuck. Having a 'trainer's box of tricks' (see page 308) may help.

  Be honest if you have to change the programme slightly because you do not have vital material. Explain this to the group, and you might find women come up with an alternative – use the group as a resource!

- *Complaints over getting started*
  Some women will fail to see why so much time is spent on the preliminaries – introductions, icebreakers, expectations, ground rules. You may need to balance this important first part with their impatience, and sometimes it is enough to tell the group why you are spending so much time. Scene-setting is particularly important if dealing with difficult issues.

- *Running out of time*
  When producing a framework, the temptation is to include everything. Be realistic about what can be achieved in the time you have. Going over-time is not helpful to crèche workers, women with children, or women who have to leave on time for whatever reasons.

  If you are not getting everything done by a certain time, check your programme, and rearrange or delete an activity. You can also explain to the group that time is a problem, and negotiate what should be done or left out.

  It is easy to arrive at the end of a session and not have time for evaluation, or to try and rush an evaluation activity. Make sure you have allowed enough time to evaluate, even if this means changing the method of evaluation to a shorter one.

- *Anger at the end of the event*
  Sometimes passions are raised, disagreements occur, emotions are shared, and women get angry. If this happens, it is useful to round off the event with a closing activity that brings women together. You cannot plan for unexpected turmoil, so have a variety of closing activities to hand (section 8) and adjust your programme accordingly.

The more experienced you become, the more you will feel confident about producing your own frameworks, and will adapt them to suit the group as you go along.

Links with other sections

Section 3: Training in women's health education
Section 4: Working with women
Section 6: Learning from experience
Section 7: Evaluation
Section 8: Running sessions/training others
Section 10: Making it happen – Opportunities for training
Section 11: General resources

Resources

Books

Alinsky, Saul. *Community organising – you've never really tried it.* Available from London Voluntary Services Council, 68 Chalton Street, London NW1 1JR. Telephone: 071 388 0241. £1.
Humorous and radical approach to community work.

Gann, Robert. *The health information handbook – resources for self-care* (1986). Gower Publishing, Aldershot. Telephone: 0252 331551. £35.
Practical and sensitive guide to self-help in health, with information and ideas which could be adapted as part of a course focusing on women gaining health knowledge for themselves.

Rodmell, Sue and Watt, Alison. *The politics of health education: raising the issues* (1986). Routledge, London. £8.95.
Collection of mainly theoretical essays but useful background to the political issues involved in health education.

Packs

Green, Felicity (ed). Health education foundation course (1990). Available from Stockport Health Promotion Unit, 188 Buxton Road, Stockport. £25.
The principles of health and adult education presented in a pack intended for use over a six-day period.

Women and health, activities and materials Health Education Council/WEA. (1986). Available from WEA North Western District, 4th Floor, Crawford House, Precinct Centre, Oxford Road, Manchester M13 9GH. £6 plus p.&p.
Very useful pack containing activities and materials for use in women's health courses and discussion groups.

Richardson, Carolyn. *Negotiating assertively* (1990). Available from Pavilion Publishing, 42 Lansdowne Place, Hove, East Sussex BN3 1HH. £32.50.
Aimed at professionals but includes useful group exercises, handouts and so on – if you can afford the price!

Scottish Health Education Group. *A guide to running courses for nurses, midwives and health visitors* (1989). Available from Health Education Board for Scotland, Woodburn House, Canaan Lane, Edinburgh EH10 4SG. Telephone: 031 447 8044. £30.
Includes guidelines on topics like sharing counselling skills, together with outlines/models of health courses.

Organisations
Open University Community Education, The Open University, Walton Hall, Milton Keynes MK7 6AA.
The Community Education faculty publishes a wide range of teaching materials on health issues – write for a catalogue.
Open University Educational Enterprises Ltd., 12 Cofferidge Close, Stony Stratford, Milton Keynes MK11 1BY. Telephone 0908 261662.
It is worth writing to this department of the Open University for their broadcast calendar. This lists all the OU radio and television programmes for the year – those related to women, health and education can be a stimulating source of ideas and information. OU Educational Enterprises also sells individual study units – the written material to accompany the broadcasts – write for details.

SECTION TEN

Making it happen – opportunities for training

	What this section contains	**262**
	How this section can be of use	**263**
	Setting the scene	**264**
10.1	ACTIVITY: back to life, back to reality	265
10.2	ACTIVITY: gaining support for training	268
	Collaborating with other organisations	
	Organisations with which to liaise	270
	Key people to contact and work with	271
	Advantages of organisations working together	271
	Interagency planning: points to remember	273
	Liaising with other organisations	273
	Training within an organisation	**274**
	Meeting your needs: relating to training events	**274**
	Case-studies: developing women's health training	**276**
	Publicity	
	Points to remember when publicising an event	277
	Who is the event for?	277
	Why women may not respond	277
	Information to send to registered participants	277
	Where will you publicise?	278
	How will you publicise?	278
	What will you publicise?	278

Samples

Publicity material	280
Registration form	282
Separate crèche form	283
Letter to be sent out on receipt of registration form	284
Co-tutor contracts	286
Calendar of religious/cultural festivals	289
Links with other sections	**291**
Resources	**291**

What this section contains

Previous sections have provided information, activities, and ideas for putting together different kinds of women's health training events, and have discussed issues around women's health work. This section looks at how to create, take up, or develop opportunities for training. It contains:

- An appraisal of the current climate for training opportunities.
- Opportunities for training either between or within organisations.
- Who to contact in statutory or voluntary organisations, or in the community.
- How training has been developed through the HEA 'Health Education for Women Training Project'.
- The practicalities of publicity.

There are no right ways to create opportunities for training – there will be huge variations between organisations in different areas, and different opportunities available throughout the country. It is a question of acknowledging and building on local possibilities. Networking is crucial.

How this section can be of use

You can use this section for yourself, or to train others. It may:

- help you to appraise your own practice in terms of taking up or promoting opportunities for training;
- give you ideas on how to go about training;
- encourage you to liaise with other organisations;
- help you to realise that obstacles to training may be due to local variations in possibilities or the reality of women's lives, not to your own lack of skill.

Setting the scene

- Opportunities for training are affected by the economic and political climate in which we live. Funding and income generation are particular issues for the NHS and the local education authorities (LEAs). Today, there is greater emphasis on self-help and personal responsibility than on collective and community development approaches.
- Access to decision-making bodies can be difficult. There can be a lack of empathy with and commitment to this way of working within formal structures.
- Because lip-service often is paid to training, there may be little appreciation of or commitment to effective training. The quality of training is often overlooked as long as it can be shown that some kind of training has taken place.
- Within the hard-pressed community education services, there are few free courses for women that are not aimed at getting them low-paid, low-status jobs or work where there are acute shortages. Voluntary adult organisations are facing funding crises and are able to offer fewer free courses.
- Expensive training often is viewed as being of higher status and quality, but there are less funds available for staff to attend.
- Managers can block information about training events reaching the staff who would benefit from it.
- Women are sometimes having to pay for their own training needs, and attend training events in their own time. This is particularly pertinent for part-time workers.
- There are local variations in health and local authority organisations. What is easy to organise in one area may prove more difficult in another. For example, there may be thriving voluntary organisations, women's groups and community groups in some places and not in others.
- The reality of women's lives needs to be taken into account. For example, for women with children consider:
  - school holidays;
  - in-service training days for teachers;
  - unexpected school closures;
  - schools, even within a geographical area, can have holidays at different times.
- Women are less likely to be in a career structure and so tend to move jobs more frequently than men. You may spend time searching out women to work with, only to find they have moved on.

- The weather can seriously affect training events. Bad weather often results in a breakdown in transport, leading to women being unable to attend planning meetings or training events.

10.1 ACTIVITY: back to life, back to reality

Aims
- To explore the limitations of putting training into practice.
- To look at good practice and planning for training events.

Materials
Flipchart paper, pens, and Worksheet (page 267) for each woman.

Method

Time: 1 hour

1. In small groups look at the Worksheet.
2. Feedback and flipchart group responses.
3. Group carousel activity, with each woman taking her most relevant point with her into the carousel.

CAROUSEL
1. After forming two circles (one inner, one outer), each woman in the outer ring has 30 seconds to state her point.
2. Each corresponding woman in the inner ring has one minute to respond with advice/empathy/information/contacts/ideas/support/similar experience.
3. Ten seconds to digest this and then to move around one until the circle is completed.
4. The inner circle now becomes the outer circle and the activity is repeated.

Possible outcomes

- Offers the chance to restate and refine the problem, as well as to receive different kinds of responses.
- Gives each woman the chance to hear from, and respond to, half the group personally.
- An economical way to get a number of ideas out and passed around.

(*continued on page 268*)

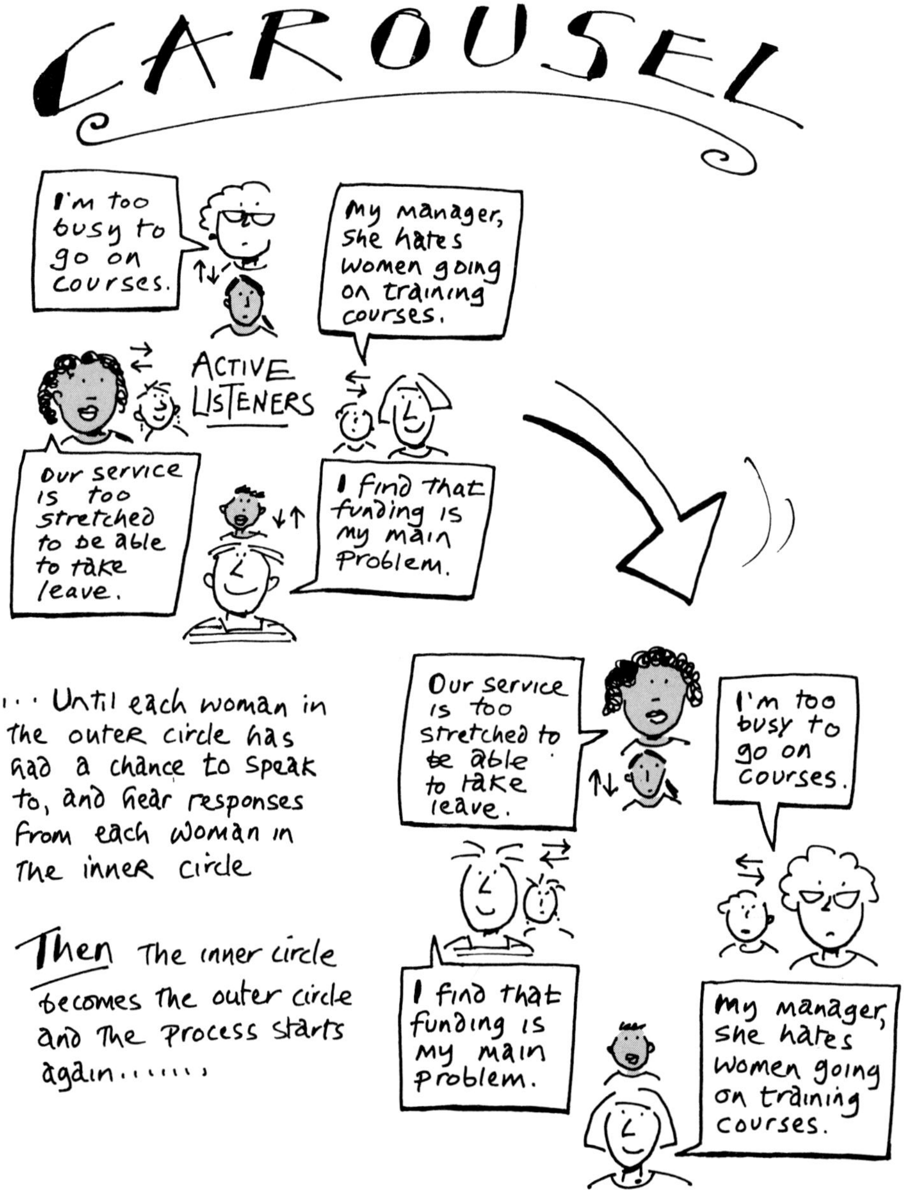
CAROUSEL
I'm too busy to go on courses.
My manager, she hates women going on training courses.
ACTIVE LISTENERS
Our service is too stretched to be able to take leave.
I find that funding is my main problem.
... Until each woman in the outer circle has had a chance to speak to, and hear responses from each woman in the inner circle
Then the inner circle becomes the outer circle and the process starts again......
Our service is too stretched to be able to take leave.
I'm too busy to go on courses.
I find that funding is my main problem.
My manager, she hates women going on training courses.

WORKSHEET: back to life, back to reality

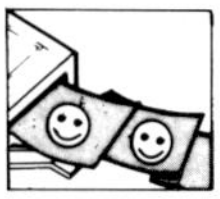

A10.1

- What do you feel could hinder you from doing this type of work in the future in both organisational and personal terms?

- Each woman choose the most relevant issue for herself.

- Women may change their perception of their problem or it may become clearer by restating it.
- Provides a balanced way of looking at limitations.

10.2 ACTIVITY: gaining support for training

Aims

- To enable women to focus on the difficulties they experience in getting support for training.
- To enable women to share possible solutions to the blocks to training they experience.

Materials

Flipchart questions (difficulties):

- What are the blocks you experience?
- How could your own behaviour hinder support for training?
- What are the basic issues regarding training that add to your difficulties?

PROMPTSHEET: questions (solutions):

- What factors may help you gain support for training?
- How could your own behaviour help?

Method **Time: 1 hour**

1. In large group, with flipchart questions prominently displayed, ask women to brainstorm responses to each question. Flipchart responses.
2. Give copy of Promptsheet to each woman. In small groups, ask women to discuss solutions to the difficulties flipcharted.
3. Report back to large group.

Possible responses

- Typical blocks to training which women experience are:
  - lack of information on what training is available;
  - no shared agreement within organisation on what constitutes 'training';
  - lack of information on actual training budget of organisation;
  - lack of training opportunities for part-time workers;
  - organisation not having strategic plan or decision-making process regarding training for employees;
  - training is often reactive: employers do not consider training until employees reveal they are not able to undertake the work expected of them;
  - work seen as having to come first: if there is a 'crisis', may be expected to drop a training event;
  - lack of cover at work while undergoing training.
- Kinds of behaviour which hinder support for training:
  - low expectation of getting support for training;
  - cynical/negative attitude;
  - being willing to pay for training yourself;
  - being willing to undertake training in your own time;
  - feeling guilty about asking for training; about going (and others having to cover for you).
- Basic issues around training which add to your difficulties:
  - lip-service being paid to training;
  - training seen as a 'one-off' rather than as a process;
  - cost of training;
  - timing of training;
  - lack of childcare facilities to enable women to participate in training.
- Factors which may help you gain support for training:
  - knowing how important training is for you, and therefore how much energy you are prepared to put into gaining support for it;
  - being clear about why you want specific training;
  - knowing the training budget for your organisation;
  - knowing how decisions are made regarding who is eligible for training;
  - being able to show management either in writing or in a meeting: that you have researched possibilities for training; detailed information regarding the specific training you are seeking; how your training will benefit the organisation; your willingness to provide feedback on what you have gained from the training;
  - being aware of what you are prepared to compromise on!

- Ways in which your behaviour could help:
  - have expectations that your training needs should be met;
  - be assertive in negotiating for what you want;
  - enlist support from colleagues.

Discussion points and issues raised

- It may be useful for women to role-play asking for training from their organisation. Rest of group could observe and make helpful suggestions.

  (Idea from Manchester Business School Women's Enterprise Unit.)

Collaborating with other organisations

Organisations with which to liaise

- National Health Service:
  - Especially district health authorities (DHAs, many of which have a training department); health promotion units; community units.
  - Family health services authorities (FHSAs) – GPs are being encouraged by FHSAs to set up health promotion clinics. These are often topic-based, but could encompass, for example, women's health discussion groups. Many health workers feel they lack groupwork skills.
  - Primary health care facilitators are being appointed by some FHSAs. Their role is to encourage the setting up of initiatives to promote positive health, especially within the community.
- Youth and community services.
- Social services.
- Probation services.
- Local Education Authority (especially community education departments)
- Voluntary adult education organisations, for example Workers Educational Associations (WEAs).
- Well-Woman Centres.
- University extra-mural departments.
- Community health councils.
- Local women's groups.

Key people to contact and work with

- Managers and in-service training officers of statutory organisations such as the NHS are useful people to liaise with regarding training around women's health. Because this may be a new way of working for them, a relationship of mutual understanding, respect, and support must first be established.
- You may find yourself liaising with someone you have worked with before or know may be interested in what you are trying to achieve. It is important to concentrate on those people who are keen and interested. If they are not in positions of management, then contact their managers or in-service training officers, if only to inform them of what you are planning to do together.
- Managers may not wish to be involved, but it is essential they are kept informed for the following reasons:
  - they may be able to offer resources and support;
  - it helps get the work integrated into existing structures – particularly important if they are training structures;
  - avoids feelings of treading on someone else's patch;
  - helps gain credibility and value for the work.
- If the key person is in a managerial position, the advantages include:
  - they may take on responsibilities as part of their ongoing work;
  - the work may receive a higher profile from the outset;
  - publicity and information-giving can be done through their channels;
  - women wishing to attend training events are more likely to be able to do so in work time.

Advantages of organisations working together

- There will be a variety of experiences, skills, and resources to draw on, especially if there are several organisations involved.
- Energy levels may be higher owing to spreading of workload.
- Women can learn from each other through direct experience.
- Publicity and information may be circulated more efficiently and comprehensively.
- If there are statutory and voluntary organisations working together, there may be mutual learning about different ways of working.

(*continued on page 273*)

Key people to contact and work with

You could talk to these people		People you might approach more formally
Health visitors District nurses Community psychiatric nurses		Community nurse managers
Practice nurses		GP practices
Community workers Women's refuge workers		Social services managers Co-ordinator
Social workers		District managers
Community education tutors		Head of community education department
WEA tutor-organisers		District secretary
Parent support group workers		LEA
Women's Institute members		Local branch chair
Council for Voluntary Services (CVS) workers	They may be managed by, or accountable to	Head of local CVS
Local councillors on committees		
LEA officers		

- Issues and structures that may affect the above:
  - NHS Act.
  - Education Reform Act.
  - Care in the Community.
  - Children's Act.
  - EC initiatives.
  - Contract culture.
  - Reorganisation of services.
  - Cuts in funding.
  - Changed priorities.
  - Having a remit to work with specific groups only (e.g. unemployed women, Black women).
  - Constitutionally not being able to be involved in women-only events.

- Barriers of experts and passive recipients may be overcome.
- Greater variety of women can be targeted and reached, thereby benefiting from the training.
- Networks may be formed for the future.

Interagency planning: points to remember

- Each member of the planning team must take responsibility for and demonstrate commitment to the training event.
- A co-tutor contract may be useful, in which specific responsibilities are made clear (page 286).
- Planning and implementation will take longer.
- Different views and methods may cause complications.
- While creating opportunities, sharing funding responsibilities can make you feel you must work in a particular way on an issue you feel doubtful about.

Liaising with other organisations

- If you do not know a manager's name, phone the switchboard and find out. It is better to write/phone specific people than address by a general title.
- Write a letter first, outlining what you want, and saying you will be phoning. When you do phone, you will be expected.
- The caretaker of a local educational establishment may be a wonderful source of useful information on who is who.
- The switchboard at, for example, the DHA or social services department, could be an excellent source of information in terms of the appropriate people to approach.
- Your local community health council may be able to advise you on who to approach within the health service or the local authority.
- Read your local newspaper regularly to gain an awareness of topical issues, organisations, and political sensitivities.

Training within an organisation

Organisations and individuals may choose to set up a training event independently.

- Advantages may include:
  - won't require lengthy planning meetings;
  - no need to compromise or make concessions to others;
  - may direct event towards specific group, topic, or issue;
  - organisers may feel more in control and benefit from the experience;
  - credit for a successful event will remain with the organisation or individual.
- Disadvantages may include:
  - resources may be scarce;
  - variety of experiences, skills, and ideas may be lacking;
  - credibility with other organisations may be more difficult to achieve;
  - the work is less likely to be taken up by other organisations (flip side of this could be that individual/organisation then retains the work);
  - fewer people will benefit from planning and participating in the event.

Meeting your needs relating to training events

If you are looking for	You could approach
someone to co-train with you	health promotion unit local Well-Woman Centre volunteers community education department social services community health council local women's group
A suitable venue	health promotion unit adult education centre health centre trade union social club community school LEA nursery school women's centre community health council

If you are looking for	You could approach
Help with producing publicity	health promotion unit community health council
Help distributing publicity	health promotion unit community health council trade union centre libraries local papers, radio local women's networks/organisations
Help with resources	health promotion unit community health council women's networks trade union centre community education department Well-Woman Centre
Funding your training event	health promotion unit district health authority regional health authority LEAs women's committees local council rural development trusts local trusts or charities Workers Educational Association
Crèche workers	crèche co-op mobile crèche local community centres under fives' project Pre-School Playgroups Association local Childminders Association social services local FE college for students doing NNEB courses local woman's organisations, for advice.

Case-studies: developing women's health training

- A health promotion officer has been allocated money for a national 'Drinkwise Day' which could be aimed at women. Instead of producing leaflets, she wishes to pay a tutor to train women in the community to run women's health groups.
- Well-Woman Centre volunteers want someone to run women's health courses within the centre to attract new volunteers. They also want someone to train the new volunteers. You offer to train them to run their own women's health sessions, and to train their own volunteers.
- Instead of working with individual health promotion officers in a geographical area, you suggest they get together and you work with them as a group. They benefit from sharing experiences, supporting each other, and learning about other district health authorities.
- Women using a local community centre have heard it may be closed by the council. You offer them training to build their confidence, learn new skills, and run women's health sessions for themselves. The council is less likely to close the centre if the women can demonstrate uses for it.
- You set up a multidisciplinary training day around the *Women and Health* pack outside of work time, targeting a large range of women from health professionals through to women's refuge workers. Women who have attended these days then go back to their workplace settings and ask for more training.
- Well-Woman campaigners want to run women and health days, with support and help as training for themselves, and to raise the profile of women's health in the community.
- You decide to convene an ongoing group of women who work with women around any health issues. You convene the first meeting but thereafter the responsibility for running the sessions rotates and is planned from session to session.
- A community education worker contacts you to run workshops in groupwork skills and women's health, for women interested in tutoring women's health sessions. You involve her in the planning of the workshops, and co-train with her, taking main responsibility. Following this you have an evaluation session together. She then feels capable of running a similar workshop in the future, co-training with someone less experienced.
- You may be able to develop training to coincide with national events that are well publicised such as 'Drinkwise Day', 'No-smoking Day', and 'World AIDS Day'.

Even Mother's Day could be an opportunity for running training events around issues such as being a mother!

Publicity

(See Publicity, page 97.)

Points to remember when publicising an event

Who is the event for?

It is important to be clear about who the event is targeted at:

- If you are aiming to attract women from different minority ethnic groups, be aware when setting dates for your event of different cultural festivals and customs that may prevent some women from attending (see page 289).
- If you want to attract women with children, you will need to offer good crèche facilities to encourage these women to come along, and avoid school holidays.

Why women may not respond

This may have nothing to do with the actual publicity, but may instead be related to:

- Lack of time – not being able to attend in work time.
- Publicity sent through managers can take ages to filter down.
- Inappropriate times (children's holidays, weekends, weekdays). It can be useful to have a section on the reply slip for women to fill in if they cannot come saying whether weekday/weekend would be better or expressing an interest in future events.
- Childcare commitments may be too great, or the crèche inappropriate.
- Too many other commitments, need to prioritise.

Information to send to registered participants

As soon as possible after the closing date for registration, send:

- Welcoming letter, including venue, date, timings of the day.
- Confirmation of crèche needs they have requested.
- List any special needs they have pointed out (state whether or not you can meet them – this can really reassure participants).
- Phone number of venue.

- If women are expected to attend the entire event, say so. Give phone numbers of facilitators just before event and ask women to let you know if they cannot come after all, which saves everyone waiting for people who are never going to turn up.
- Map of venue, bus/parking details.
- List of participants. It can be useful to say a bit about them, but avoid professional titles. This is particularly important for multidisciplinary events where voluntary workers can feel intimidated by professionals. Also, titles often fail to give an idea of the work women actually do around women's health.

Where will you publicise?

- Do you wish wide or limited circulation of publicity?
- If you publicise widely, will you be able to cope with the possible response?
- Word-of-mouth can be a successful means of publicity, but can exclude some women.

How will you publicise?

- Local radio? Local newspaper? A 'tame' reporter on the local rag can be very useful, but it is essential to give accurate and adequate information.
- The above is not a useful way of publicising if you need women to register in advance. If you are not asking for pre-registration, difficulties can be encountered through over-attendance, or non-attendance, at the event.
- Leaflets, through networks/community health councils/direct mailing/public venues.
- Posters, through networks/public places, for example libraries.

What will you publicise?
Leaflets and posters should be *clear and concise, with the vital information prominent* (*and accessible to your audience in terms of language, style, and availability*):

- Title of event.
- Date, time, place of event.
- Aims of the event.
- Costs of the event.

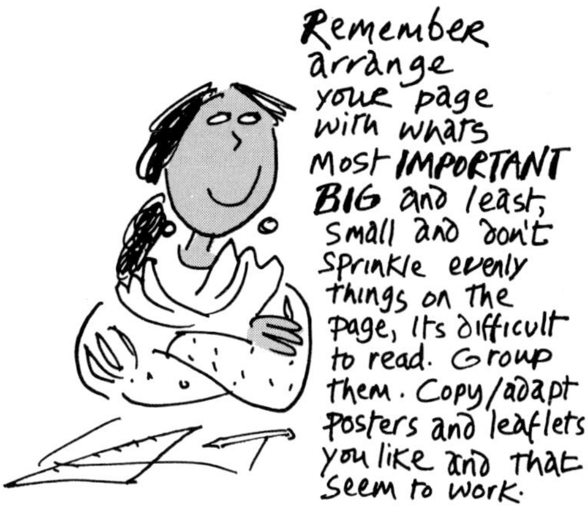
Remember arrange your page with whats most IMPORTANT BIG and least, small and don't sprinkle evenly things on the page, its difficult to read. Group them. Copy/adapt posters and leaflets you like and that seem to work.

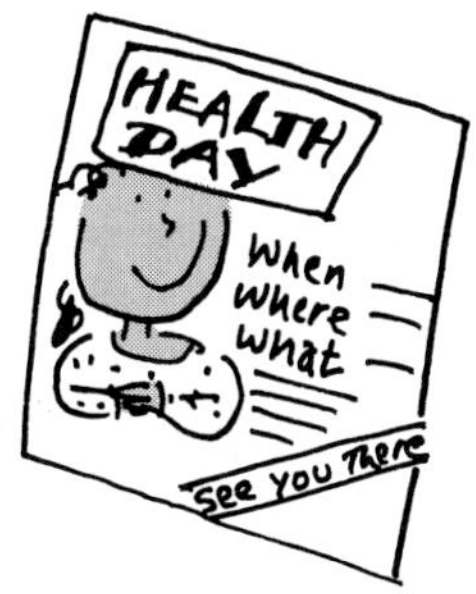
HEALTH DAY
When
Where
What
See you there

- Practicalities: time; crèche; lunch; access.
- Organisation/key person to contact (address/phone number).
- State whether women need to attend the entire event.

Leaflets *with registration slips should include:*

- Reply-by date.
- Address for return.
- A section for participants to state their particular interest in the event.
- A section for participants to state their experience in women's health.
- Childcare requirements (including special needs).
- Any special needs.
- Section for name, address, and phone number.

This information can help you plan the event to suit the expressed needs of the participants.

Samples of publicity material

HEALTH EDUCATION FOR WOMEN TRAINING PROJECT

TRAINING EVENTS

* ASSERTIVENESS AND HEALTH CHOICES
* WOMEN AND AIDS: THE ISSUES
* ISSUES IN TRAINING IN HEALTH EDUCATION

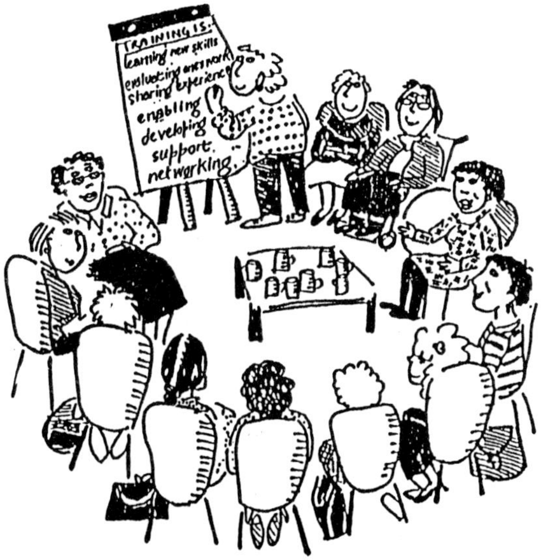
TRAINING IS:
learning new skills
sharing experience
enabling
developing
support.
networking.

STAYING HEALTHY:

WOMEN MAKING CHANGES

HEALTH EDUCATION AUTHORITY

WORKERS EDUCATIONAL ASSOCIATION

WORKERS EDUCATIONAL ASSOCIATION

HEALTH EDUCATION FOR WOMEN TRAINING PROJECT

WOMEN AND HIV/AIDS:

ISSUES IN HEALTH EDUCATION

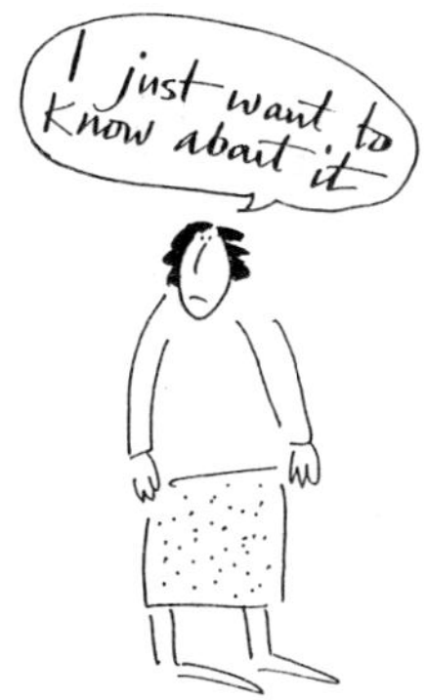
I just want to know abait it

STAYING HEALTHY:

WOMEN MAKING CHANGES

HEALTH EDUCATION AUTHORITY

WORKERS EDUCATIONAL ASSOCIATION

WOMEN & HEALTH COURSE

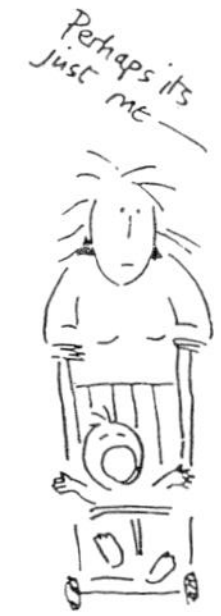
Perhaps its just me

* WHERE: BISHOP MASKELL CENTRE, LOWER GALDEFORD, LUDLOW

* WHEN: TUESDAYS, 10.00 A.M. - 2.00 P.M.

* STARTING DATE: 27th June, 1989 for 3 weeks

* FOR MORE DETAILS CONTACT:

JENNY on Ludlow 890665 or
CHRIS on Leominster 4224

Come to this informal discussion group to look at some of the main health issues that affect women's lives. There will be plenty of time to ask questions and share experiences. Topics will be decided by the group but will probably include:

* Period problems and pre-menstrual tension
* Stress, depression and relaxation
* Problems such as cystitis and thrush
* Alternative forms of medicine
* How to be a mother and stay sane!
* Breast and cervical cancer
* Eating more healthily, dieting
* Menopause and ageing

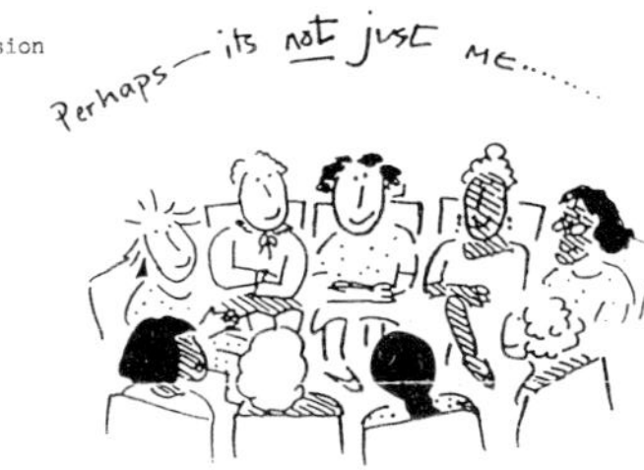
Perhaps — its not just me......

WOMEN OF ALL AGES WELCOME

COST: FREE
BRING LUNCH TO SHARE
CHILDCARE AVAILABLE

ORGANISED BY THE WORKERS' EDUCATIONAL ASSOCIATION

Samples

Example of a registration form

(name and date(s) of event)

Please PRINT clearly

YOUR NAME ....

ADDRESS (for mailing) ....

....

.... Postcode ....

Tel: .... (day) .... (evening)

DO YOU NEED THE CRÈCHE? yes/no

No. of children age(s) ....

Any special requirements ....

....

HAVE YOU ANY SPECIAL NEEDS? yes/no

Please say what they are ....

....

....

MEALS

Vegetarian/vegan/other (please explain)

....

The following sections will enable us to plan the event more closely to your needs

WHAT IS YOUR INTEREST IN THIS EVENT? INCLUDE WORK IF RELEVANT

....

....

PARTICULAR ISSUES YOU WOULD LIKE COVERED

....

....

....

Please return this slip by .... (date) ....

to: ....

Example of a separate crèche form (particularly useful for a longer event)

Please use a separate form for each child you are bringing

NAME OF CHILD ....

AGE ....

BOY/GIRL ....

ADDRESS ....

....

MOTHER'S NAME ....

IF ENGLISH IS NOT YOUR CHILD'S FIRST LANGUAGE, DOES S/HE NEED SOMEONE TO HELP THEM WITH LANGUAGE?

yes/no

If yes, which language? ....

FOOD

Any special diet? ....

HEALTH

Is there anything the crèche workers should be aware of?

....

TOILET

nappy/potty/toilet (delete those not applicable)

SLEEP

needed/not needed

cot/mattress

what time does your child usually have a sleep? ....

PLEASE TICK IF YOU DO NOT WISH YOUR CHILD TO BE LOOKED AFTER BY A MALE CRÈCHE WORKER ☐

ANYTHING ELSE YOU WOULD LIKE CRÈCHE WORKERS TO KNOW?

....

....

(continued)

(Sample crèche form, continued)

I AGREE TO MY CHILD GOING ON THE ORGANISED OUTING yes/no
Name .... Signature ....

Please return this form by .... (date)..................
to: ....

Please bring a change of clothing in a bag with the child's name on. If bringing a favourite toy, please label!

Example of letter to be sent out on receipt of registration form

Date
Address

Dear ....

EVENT/DATE(S)/VENUE

Thank you for returning your completed registration form for the above event.

The event will be held at (full address of venue)
Time
(include parking and bus details)

Your particular needs have been noted. These are . . . (list from completed registration form)

CRÈCHE ....
SPECIAL NEEDS ....
MEALS ....

(If you need women to wear special clothing, for example for relaxation session, say so in this letter.)

(continued)

(letter, continued)

(If you have indicated on the publicity that women should bring packed lunch, remind them now.)

We are assuming that, since you have registered, you are able to attend the entire event.

If you do *not* need the crèche after all, please tell us. If you find you *cannot* come after all, please let us know. This saves us waiting for women who are not going to turn up. (Name) can be contacted at (Tel. no.) up to (date/time). The telephone number of the venue is ....

If you have any other queries about the event, please contact (names/phone nos).

We look forward to seeing you.

Enclosures:

- map of venue;
- list of other women coming/what area (or job) they come from.

Examples of co-contracts

If you are working with someone else, it is important to be clear at the outset how you will work together by

- organising the event;
- running the event;
- evaluating the event.

Example of a co-contract for organising the event

EVENT details

AIMS OF THE EVENT

FUNDING THE EVENT

KEY WORKERS

ROLES OF KEY WORKERS

- first worker
  (for example,
  publicity ....
  write up notes of meeting ....
  organise crèche ....)
  meet with second worker on .... basis
  time available for organising ....

- second worker
  (for example,
  sort out venue ....
  obtain refreshments ....
  get hold of video equipment ....)
  meet with first worker on .... basis
  time available for organising ....

Example of a co-contract for running the event (especially useful if more than two women are leading the event, and for a longer event)

Co-tutor(s) (trainer(s)/facilitator(s))

....

....

....

....

Lead responsibility for different parts of the programme

name .... session ....

....

....

....

- We will meet during the event:
  - to revise rest of programme as necessary;
  - to give feedback on sessions;
  - to support each other.
- We all have equal responsibility for the success of the event.
- We want to learn from each other.
- We have different ways of facilitating.
- If we are not happy with the way each of us facilitates, we are free to say so (in the spirit of constructive criticism).
- We will meet *after* the event to evaluate, and look at ways of building on the event.

Example of a co-contract to evaluate each other

This can be a tool to improve the style and practice of each co-tutor ....

- Did we work as a team?
- Did we stick to our programme of who was taking lead responsibility for each session?
- Did we share responsibility for the event?
- What were the *advantages* of co-tutoring this event?
- What were the *disadvantages* of co-tutoring this event?
- What did each of us do well?
- What could each of us have done better?
- Were there times when each of us was too active/talkative/directive?
- Were there times when each of us was too passive/non-directive?
- What did each of us learn from tutoring this event?
- Did the event highlight any further training needs for ourselves?

Calendar of religious/cultural festivals

Festivals are important in different cultures and religions. Whilst festivals can be marked with a feast day, a celebration, they are often combined with a sense of solemnity and dedication. Fasting often comes before having a feast. Some major festivals require absence from school or work.

It is for these reasons that it is important to be aware of where in the calendar different festivals occur which will be relevant to the particular women you are aiming your event at.

Organising a two-day residential event to include Muslim women in the middle of the fasting month of Ramadan would not be an ideal time, for example.

The following is a calendar of some religious festivals, showing which month they took place in 1991. It is *only a guide*, since the dates of so many festivals will vary from year to year because calendars are different in various parts of the world. Muslim festivals fall 11–12 days earlier each year. The Muslim day begins in the evening and depends on actually seeing the new moon.

For an up-to-date calendar of festivals, contact:

National Society for Religious Education Centre (NSREC)
23 Kensington Square
London W8 5HN
Tel: 071 937 4241

Cost: £2.50 (including postage)
cheques/postal orders made out to *SHAP Working Party*.

See page 290 for examples of some religious festivals.

Some religious festivals: guide for 1991

February	Yuan Tan (New Year)	Chinese
	Holi (spring harvest)	Hindu
March	Ramadan (one month fasting)	Muslim
	Good Friday	Christian
	Passover (8 days, to celebrate deliverance from Egypt of children of Israel)	Jewish
April	Baisakhi (New Year)	Sikh
	Id-ul-Fitr (feast marking the end of Ramadan)	Muslim
May	Shavuot (thanks for receiving the Torah)	Jewish
June	Martyrdom of Guru Arjan Dev	Sikh
	Id-ul-Adha (4 days, end of pilgrimage to Mecca)	Muslim
July	Al Hijrah (New Year)	Muslim
	Tisha B'av (commemorating destruction of the Temples)	Jewish
September	Rosh Hashanah (New Year)	Jewish
	Yom Kippur (holiest day, confessing sins ready for a fresh start)	Jewish
	Sukkot (8 days, harvest festival)	Jewish
October	Simchat Torah (giving thanks for the Torah)	Jewish
	Navratra (fasting and penance)	Hindu
November	Diwali (New Year festival of light)	Hindu
	Birthday of Guru Nanak Dev	Sikh
December	Hanukah (8-day festival of light)	Jewish
	Martyrdom of Guru Tegh Bahadur	Sikh
	Christmas Day	Christian

Links with other sections

Section 6: Learning from experience

Resources

see also: General resources section 11
other materials on planning and organising under Resources in section 8 and section 6

Books

Allen, Rosemary and Purkis, Andrew. *Health in the round: voluntary action and antenatal services* (1983). Bedford Square Press. £4.95.
Although primarily concerned with antenatal services, this book gives useful guidelines on working in partnership with the statutory sector, with excellent examples of good practices.

Birch, Carrie and Houghton, Nina. *The ABC of Crèche Training*. Available from Daycare Trust, Wesley House, 4 Wild Court, London WC2B 5AU. £4.55.
Excellent guide to running a crèche – including training, funding, publicity, and evaluation. Many of the guidelines could be adapted for other kinds of training courses, but it is also invaluable for anyone who has to consider childcare needs of women on courses.

Bowman, Marion and Norte, M. *Raising money for women – a survivor's guide* (1986). Bedford Square Press. Available from NCVO, Regents Wharf, 8 All Saints Street, London N1 9RL. £5.95.

Davison, Ann and Seary, Bill. *Grants from Europe* (1990). Bedford Square Press. £7.95.
Advice on raising money and influencing policy in Europe, which could be helpful for women involved in long-term training projects which may be eligible for European funding.

Developing partnerships between self-help groups and health promoters. Available from National Self-Help Group, 26 Bedford Square, London WC1B 3HU. Telephone: 071 636 4066. £4.

Drinkwater, Jane. *Get it on: a practical guide to getting airtime* (1984). Pluto, London. Everything you need to know about getting radio publicity.

Fieldgrass, J. *Partnerships in health promotion: collaboration between the statutory and voluntary sectors* (1992). Health Education Authority. Available from the HEA, Hamilton House, Mabledon Place, London WC1H 9TX. £11.

Gawlinski, G. and Graessle, L. *Planning together: the art of effective teamwork* (1988). Bedford Square Press. £9.95.

Holloway, Christine and Otto, Shirley. *Getting organised: a handbook for non-statutory organisations* (1985). Bedford Square Press. Available from NCVO, Regents Wharf, 8 All Saints Street, London N1 9RL. £4.95.

National Council for Voluntary Organisations. *Finding funds: general information on funding for voluntary groups* (1991). Available from NCVO, Regents Wharf, 8 All Saints Street, London N1 9RL. Telephone: 071 636 4066. £4.
Concise guidelines on all aspects of fundraising, especially useful for small groups.

NCVO. *Partners in learning: voluntary/statutory collaboration in adult education* (1990). Available from Local Voluntary Action Department, NCVO, Regents Wharf, 8 All Saints Street, London N1 9RL. £3.

Organising health events for women (1991). Health Education Authority. Available from HEA, Hamilton House, Mabledon Place, London WC1H 9TX. £2.95.

Purton, Rowland. *Festivals and celebrations* (1989). Basil Blackwell. £7.50.
A comprehensive collection of festivals and celebrations drawn from all the world's religions. Very useful.

Organisations

Daycare Trust/National Childcare Campaign, Wesley House, 4 Wild Court, London WC2B 5AU. Telephone: 071 405 5617.
Information on local information services for children and also publish a quarterly newsletter (£1.50 per copy) on all aspects of childcare.

Rural Unit, NCVO, Regents Wharf, 8 All Saints Street, London N1 9RL.
The Rural Unit publishes a range of leaflets of special interest to those working in rural areas, on topics like community care, networking, planning, and partnerships.

Voluntary Organisations Liaison Council for Under Fives, 77 Holloway Road, London N7 8JZ.
Useful source of information and resources for parents with young children. Hire a video *My mum thinks she's funny* on services offered by voluntary organisations. £20 to rent for a week, including ten copies of booklet.

SECTION ELEVEN

General resources

This section provides a guide to resources which may be useful. It can be frustrating if you can neither find nor afford books, packs, films, or the like that you feel are essential. Do not forget that ideas and activities can be adapted – so it is worth looking at resources on training or adult education, even if they are not concerned with either women or health! Talk to as many people as you can about your plans – making links or 'networking' can be as useful for ideas as the best training handbook.

Local resources

Library

Useful for local information, as a place to publicise your event, and for training and health information resources. Books are classified according to subject. You can ask a librarian for help or you may find useful books under Education, Psychology, Health and Medicine. Some libraries have special sections, for example, Women, Gay and Lesbian, Afro-Caribbean, Asian, and so on. All libraries have a reference section which includes dictionaries and directories. Some libraries also lend videos. Although many of the videos on health are not very good, a 'bad' video can still be useful as a starting point for discussion. Borrowing books and videos from libraries is free. Libraries can often get books they do not stock from other branches – but this usually takes a long time, so plan ahead.

Phone books

The phone book and/or the Yellow Pages have the numbers of your local authority, health authority, and so on – usually with the different departments listed. Neighbourhood offices and other local services are often listed in the yellow pages under 'local government' or 'government offices'. Doctors are listed under 'medical practitioners'. The phone book is also useful when planning publicity – health centres may be listed under 'clinics', look under 'leisure' for places offering keep fit, weight training, swimming, and so on. For referring women on, Rape Crisis and the Samaritans are also listed in the phone book.

Citizens Advice Bureau (CAB)
Provides free information and advice to individuals on all subjects, for example on local resources, social security, housing, welfare, legal issues, consumer rights, and so on. They are a good source of information on how such organisations as the council, health authority and social services work. They produce a range of videos and publications on welfare issues such as benefits, debt, and on training skills, mainly aimed at advice workers. Prices, as well as the address of your local CAB, can be obtained from NACAB, Myddelton House, 115–123 Pentonville Road, London N1 9LZ. Tel. 071 833 2181.

Community Health Councils (CHCs)
These represent the health concerns of the local community and provide a consumer voice to health authorities. CHCs can provide information about the availability of women doctors, Well-Woman Clinics, and other services. Many CHCs campaign on health service provision; one example is the availability of family planning clinics. Some produce local guidelines to using the health services. CHCs vary a great deal but it is worth contacting your local one to see if they can offer information, support or publicity. The Association of Community Health Councils, 30 Drayton Park, London N5 1PB. Tel. 071 609 8405 can tell you where your nearest CHC is.

Health promotion/health education units (HPUs)
These units initiate a wide range of health promotion/education projects. They provide support, training, and resources for workers in the statutory and voluntary sectors, and in the community. They may employ people with special responsibility for working in the community, with women, ethnic minorities, older people, or people with disabilities. HPUs may be able to offer resources such as partnership in a project; they may have or be prepared to buy health education packs which can be used by local groups. Examples of projects with which they may be involved include 'smoke stop support', 'Look After Your Heart', stress management, better use of leisure facilities, and encouraging local restaurants/work canteens to offer healthy food. HPUs may be based with district health authorities, or with local authorities (in the department of environmental health). They are in the telephone book under the health authority or the council, or ask at the library, the CHC or a Well-Woman Centre. Theoretically, all HPUs are committed to the World Health Organisation's 'Health for All' declaration, so it is worth asking your HPU what it is doing for women and suggesting that it supports women's initiatives.

Well-Woman Centres/clinics
The term 'well woman' now covers many things, from an all male general practice

which offers cervical smears, to a health centre staffed by women and offering everything from family planning to aromatherapy.

Well-Woman Centres tend to be self-help centres within the community, running 'drop ins', stocking information, running courses, and offering counselling and advice. They usually cannot give any medical advice. They may be able to help with training materials, a place to meet, moral support and knowledge, and experience of women's health concerns. Staff may even be prepared to contribute their skills or time to a training course. It is worth bearing in mind that most Well-Woman Centres are under-resourced themselves.

Well-Woman clinics tend to be part of either health authority or GP provision, offering a session with a doctor or health worker for cervical smears and routine screening.

You can find out if you have a local Well-Woman Centre or clinic from the library, the CHC, or the family planning clinic. They are often listed in the telephone book under 'clinics'.

Councils for Voluntary Service (CVS)
Provide support and encourage voluntary action. They may have paid staff or be run by volunteers and depending on their resources, can offer use of office facilities, help with funding applications, local information, meeting rooms, and so on. Look in your phone book for your local CVS.

Adult education institutes/WEA/extra-mural departments
These run a wide range of courses during the day and in the evening, usually at a low cost. If you do not have the resources or premises to run a women's health course yourself, you could approach your local adult education institute and offer to teach one – often, if there are enough people prepared to do the course (usually at least 12), they will consider putting one on. The Workers Educational Association (WEA) runs courses in many parts of the country and also produces a women's education publication list, as well as other packs and resources aimed at women. They are available from WEA, 17 Victoria Park Square, Bethnal Green, London E2 9PB. Extra-mural departments are part of universities or polytechnics offering courses, conferences, and other educational events to the general public. In some places they are very active and accessible, holding events like 'The Politics of Women's Health', lecture series, interesting speakers, and so on. They are also likely to have expensive equipment like videos, slide projectors, and microphones. If you live near a university or polytechnic, it is worth phoning to see what they do and if they would welcome input/partnership, or could offer any resources.

Directories

Most directories are expensive, but they are often available in libraries or you could ask the health promotion unit, social services or adult education to consider buying those which would be useful to everyone.

Bradford, Nikki. *The Well-Woman's self-help directory* (1990). Sidgwick and Jackson. £12.99.
Comprehensive listing of self-help resources, alternative medical practitioners and wide range of options for women taking action on health.

Centre for Policy on Ageing. *Directory of services for elderly people in the UK* (1990). Longman. £32. Available from CPA, 25–31 Ironmonger Row, London EC1Y 3QP. Tel. 071 253 1787.

Charities Aid Foundation. *Give as you earn directory of charities* (1990). Charities Aid Foundation, 48 Pembury Road, Tunbridge, Kent TN9 2JD.
Comprehensive list of British charities and their aims.

Charities Aid Foundation. *Directory of grant making trusts.* List of trusts/foundations offering money to charities, with full details of who specialises in what, for example, animals, children, and so on. Published annually by CAF, 48 Pembury Road, Tunbridge, Kent TN9 2JD.

Church of England, General Synod. *Social responsibility: a directory of resources in the Church of England* (1987). £5.35. Available from Board for Social Responsibility, General Synod, Great Smith Street, London SW1P 3NZ.
This is currently being updated – phone 071 222 9011 and ask for Debbie Cunningham in Board for Social Responsibility for details.

Darnbrough, A. and Kinrade, D. *Directory for disabled people* (1988). RADAR (Royal Association for Disability and Rehabilitation), Cambridge.

Directory of British associations (1990). Kent, CBD.
Complete list of all voluntary organisations, mutual aid and friendly societies.

Directory of Social Change is a provider of information and training for the voluntary sector, and produces a range of publications. Contact: The Directory of Social Change, Northern Office, Federation House, Hope Street, Liverpool L1 9BW. Tel. 051 708 0117 for details.

The Everywoman directory 1991–2; women's businesses, networks and campaigns. Available from bookshops at £5.95, or mail order (£6.50) from Everywoman Publishing Ltd., 34 Islington Green, London N1 8DU.

Institute of Health Services Management. *The hospitals and health services year book.* Very detailed listing of hospitals and health services in every region, broken down by department, unit, and so on.

Loader, Leslie. *Counselling and psychotherapy resources directory* (1990). British Association of Counselling, 37a Sheep Street, Rugby, Warwickshire CV21 3BX.
Includes regional lists of individuals and organisations offering counselling.

London Voluntary Services Council. *African, Caribbean and Asian trainers directory* (1990). £3.50. Available from Central Services, LVSC, 68 Chalton Street, London NW1 1JR.
Details of trainers around the country with skills in career development, stress, mental health, alcohol, drugs, sexuality, and training.

Macdonald, Fiona. *The health directory* (1990). Thames Help/Bedford Square Press.
Directory of organisations concerned with all aspects of health, including self-help and support groups.

National Association of Local Government Women's Committees. *Directory of Women's Committees* (1990). £4.95. Available from NALGWC, The Pankhurst Centre, 60–62 Nelson Street, Manchester M13 9WP. Tel. 061 274 3684.
Invaluable guide to over 60 local authority women's committees – including details of membership, meetings, women's units, equal opportunity policies, etc.

National Council of Voluntary Organisations. *Voluntary agencies directory* (1991). Bedford Square Press, 26 Bedford Square, London WC1B 3HU.

Newton, Dorothy, Kirkwood, Janey and Lunn, Stuart (eds). *The FIAC directory of independent advice centres* (1990). £3.50. Available from Federation of Independent Advice Centres, 4th Floor, Concourse House, Lime Street, Liverpool L1 1NY.
Regional listing of advice centres in Wales, Scotland, England and Northern Ireland, including information on such things as language, availability of interpreters, and wheelchair access.

Scottish Council for Voluntary Organisations. *Directory of national voluntary organisations for Scotland* (1990). £7.50. Available from SCVO, 18–19 Claremont Crescent, Edinburgh EH7 4D. Tel. 031 556 3882.

Social services year book. This is published annually by Longman and should be held in all libraries.

Books and packs

General

A women's health bibliography. £2. Available from TUCRIC, 1st Floor, Market Buildings, Vicar Lane, Leeds LS3 7JF.

National Community Health Resource. *NCHR bibliography No. 2: evaluation* (1991). £3.95. Available from NCHR, 57 Chalton Street, London NW1 1HU.
A bibliography is a list of books on a particular topic – this one lists practical and theoretical publications on all aspects of evaluation, with details of costs and availability.

National Community Health Resource. *NCHR bibliography: selected references on black and minority ethnic health issues* (1990). £2.50. Available from NCHR, 57 Chalton Street, London NW1 1HU.

Preston, Barbara (ed). *Guide to the social services* (1990). Family Welfare Association London. £10.95. Available from Family Welfare Association, 501–5 Kingsland Road, Dalston, London E8 4AU. Tel. 071 254 6251.

Robertson, Sally (ed). *Disability rights handbook*, 16th edition April 1991–1992. Disability Alliance. £4.50. Available from Disability Alliance, Universal House, 88–94 Wentworth Street, London E1 7SA. Tel. 071 247 8776.

Smith, Caroline, *Community based health initiatives: a handbook for voluntary groups* (1982). Bedford Square Press, London.

Woollett, Stephen. *Alternative rural services* (1982). Bedford Square Press.
Encouraging and practical guide to taking action in rural areas, with a special emphasis on coping with the closure of rural facilities, for example, pharmacies, doctors' surgeries, bus services, and so on.

Training

Community Education Training Unit. *Training and how to enjoy it* (1989). £4.65. Available from CETU, Trinity Royd Cottage, Blackwall, Halifax HX1 2EH. Tel. 0422 357394.

Community Education Training Unit. *Assertion and how we train ourselves* (1990). £6.70. Available from CETU, Trinity Royd Cottage, Blackwall, Halifax HX1 2EH. Tel. 0422 357394.

Federation of Community Work Training Groups. *Learning for action: community work and participative training* (1990). Association of Metropolitan Authorities. £12.50. Available from CWTG, 356 Glossop Road, Sheffield S10 2HW.

Green, F. (ed). *Health promotion foundation course: a course for health educators on the principles and practice of health education* (1990). Stockport HPU. £25. Available from Stockport Centre for Health Education, Lyndhurst, 188 Buxton Road, Stockport SK2 7EA. Tel. 061 456 0908.

HEC/WEA *Women and health: activities and materials for use in women's health courses and discussion groups* (1986). £6 + £1.50 p.p. Available from WEA, 4th Floor, Crawford House, Precinct Centre, Oxford Road, Manchester M13 9GH. Tel. 061 273 7652.

Sapin, K. and Watters, G. *Learning from each other: a handbook for participative learning and community work learning programmes* (1990). William Temple Foundation. £14.95 + p.p. Available from William Temple Foundation, Manchester Business School, Manchester M15 6PB.

Scottish Health Education Group. *Counselling skills: a training manual* (1989). Available from Health Education Board for Scotland, Woodburn House, Canaan Lane, Edinburgh EH10 4SG.

Slavin, H. (ed). *Greater expectations: a source book for working with girls and young women* (1986). LDA Bookshops.

Smith, M. *The best is yet to come: a workbook for the middle years* (1989). Lifeskills Publishing. £12.95. Clarendon Chambers, 51 Clarendon Road, Leeds LS2 9NZ. Tel. 0532 467128.

Trainers handbook for multiracial health care (1987). £75. Available from National Extension College, 18 Brooklands Avenue, Cambridge CB2 2HN. Tel. 0223 316644.
An excellent training resource consisting of:

- Handbook (covering topics such as racism, patterns of illness, caring for people in the community, services, communication skills).
- Activities book (over 65 activities and numerous handouts which can be photocopied and used by trainers).
- Hair care supplement.

Education

Gale, P. and Purdey, M. *The adult education and training manual* (1989). Each volume £29.50. Volume 1: the adult learner and learning environment; volume 2: resourcing and organising adult learning. Available from Framework Press, St. Leonards House, St. Leonardgate, Lancaster LA1 1NN. Tel. 0524 39602.

Rogers, J. *Adults learning*. Open University Press. £6.99. Available from bookshops.

WEA. *Working towards change* (1986). Available from WEA, 17 Victoria Park Square, Bethnal Green, London E2 9PB. £5.95.
A training pack for tutors in women's education.

Women's health
HEC/WEA. *Women and health: activities and materials* (1986). £6 + £1.50 p.p. Available from WEA, 4th Floor, Crawford House, Precinct Centre, Oxford Road, Manchester M13 9GH. Tel. 061 273 7652.

Mosse, J. and Heaton, J. *The fertility and contraception book*. Faber & Faber (1990). £7.99. Available from bookshops.

Phillips, A. and Rakusen, J. (eds). *The new our bodies ourselves* (1989). Penguin Books. £12.99. Available from bookshops.

O'Sullivan, S. *Women's health: a spare rib reader* (1987). Pandora. £4.95. Available from bookshops.

Shapiro, J. (ed). *Ourselves growing older: women ageing with knowledge and power*. Fontana/Collins. £9.99. Available from bookshops.

see also
Bradford, N. *The well woman's self-help directory* under 'Directories'.

Childcare
Birch, C. and Houghton, N. *The ABC of crèche training*. £3.95. Available from Daycare Trust, Wesley House, 4 Wild Court, London WC2B 5AU.

Commission for Racial Equality. *From cradle to school: a practical guide to race equality and childcare*. Available from CRE, Elliot House, 10–12 Allington Street, London SW1E 5EH.

Orton, C. *Starting a crèche: a guide for local community groups*. Available from Gingerbread, 35 Wellington Street, London WC2E 7BN. Tel. 071 240 0953.

Organising/managing
Broady, M. and Hedley, R. *Working partnerships: community development in local authorities*. Bedford Square Press. Available from bookshops £6.95.

Health Education Authority. *Organising health events for women* (1991). £2.95 + p.&p. Available from HEA, Hamilton House, Mabledon Place, London WC1H 9TX.

Merritt, S. *Just about managing: a guide to effective management for voluntary organisations and community groups.* £7.50. Available from LVSC, 68 Chalton Street, London NW1 1JR.

Open University. *Better meetings: a handbook for individuals, groups and trainers.* Available from Learning Materials Sales Office, PO Box 188, Open University, Walton Hall, Milton Keynes MK7 6DH.

Willis, L. and Daisley, J. *Springboard: women's development workbook.* Hawthorn Press. £14.50. Available from bookshops.

Wilson, J. *Self-help groups: getting started, keeping going.* Longman. (1986).

Films and videos

CFL Vision, P.O. Box 35, Wetherby, Yorkshire LS23 7EX. Tel. 0937 541010.
Health videos for hire, some are free (with a deposit), others range from £12–30. Write for catalogue.

Cinema of Women, Unit 313, 31 Clerkenwell Close, London EC1 0AJ. Tel. 071 251 4978/081 399 5266.
Catalogue of titles stocked, price £5.

Circles, Women's Film & Video Distribution, 113 Roman Road, London E2 0HU. Tel. 071 981 6828.
Circles stock a wide range of films and videos on women and health including PMS, anorexia, mental illness, alcohol, black women and invisibility, and so on. Catalogue costs £6.50 and film/video hire ranges from £10 upwards.

Concord Films Council Limited, 201 Felixstowe Road, Ipswich, Suffolk IP3 9BJ. Tel. 0473 726012.
Stockist of Channel 4 films and videos.

Graves Medical Audio-Visual Library, Holly House, 220 New London Road, Chelmsford, Essex CM2 9BJ. Tel. 0245 283351.
Videos for sale and for hire (approx £12+VAT for 28 days) on topics such as screening, breast self-exam, and mammography.

Women's Media Resource Project, 85 Kingsland High Street, London E8 2PB. Tel. 071 254 6536.
Stocks films and videos by women – send sae for details.

Bookshops (mail order books)

Gay's the Word, 66 Marchmont Street, London WC1N 1AB. Tel. 071 278 7654.
Specialists in books of interest to lesbian women, including lesbian health.

National Extension College, 18 Brooklands Avenue, Cambridge CB2 2HN. Tel. 0223 316644.
NEC runs correspondence courses on many different topics and also publishes many books and packs of interest to people working in adult education, which are useful as resources for groups. Write for publications list/catalogue.

Silver Moon Women's Bookshop, 68 Charing Cross Road, London WC2.
All types of books of interest to women and will also order any book required.

Sisterwrite, 190 Upper Street, London N1.
Feminist bookshop stocking women's health books.

Women's Press Bookclub, 34 Great Sutton Street, London EC1V 0DX.
The bookclub offers substantial discounts on a wide range of books of special interest to women, membership costs £7.50 per year. The Women's Press at the same address sells books by mail order, send an sae for catalogue.

Organisations

The following are a selection of national organisations or networks that can put you in touch with local health/education/women's groups and/or that provide health related resources, for example, information sheets.

Action with Communities in Rural England (ACRE), Stable Yard Cottage, Fairford Park, Gloucestershire GL7 4JQ.

Association of Community Workers, Grindon Lodge, Beech Grove Road, Newcastle upon Tyne NE4 6RS. Tel. 091 272 4341.
Membership organisation for people involved in paid or unpaid community work. Fees on a sliding scale from £5–£40.

Audio Visual Training Trust, 30 Stonehouse Park, Thursby, Carlisle CA5 6NS. Tel. 0228 710712.
Offers courses in sign language, training packages and videos, and advice and information on making training accessible to deaf people. Ann Verney at AVTT can also provide details of a new and unique Deaf Women's Health Project, which aims to produce videos and leaflets in British Sign Language.

Cancerlink, 17 Britannia Street, London WC1.
An information service on all aspects of cancer, also publishes leaflets and provides special support and assistance to self-help and support groups for cancer sufferers and their friends and families.

Centre for Policy on Ageing, 25–31 Ironmonger Row, London EC1Y 3QP.
Produces wide range of publications on policy issues concerning older people, including mental illness, education, pensions, residential care, transport, and civil liberties. Aimed mainly at professionals and academics. Write with sae for a publications list.

Charity Commission, St Albans House, 57–60 Haymarket, London, SW1Y 4QX.
Official body regulating charities – groups hoping to gain charitable status have to apply to the Charity Commission.

Community Projects Foundation, 60 Highbury Grove, London N5 2AG. Tel. 071 226 5375.

Disablement Information and Advice Lines (DIAL) UK, Park Lodge, St. Catherine's Hospital, Tickhill Road, Balby, Doncaster, South Yorkshire DN4 8QN. Tel. 0302 310123. DIAL also publishes fact sheets on access, housing and education for people with disabilities (free with sae).

Family Planning Association, 27–35 Mortimer Street, London W1N 7RJ. Tel. 071 636 7866.
Provides information on local family planning clinics, free leaflets on all aspects of family planning and booklets (30p each, send sae) on premenstrual tension, self-exam, sexual difficulties, and infertility. Write for their catalogue.

Federation of Independent Advice Centres, Concourse House, Lime Street, Liverpool L1 1NY. Tel. 051 709 7444.
Network of wide range of local groups involved in some form of advice giving, for example, women's groups, youth groups, unemployment centres, women's refuges, and so on. Publishes annual directory and range of training material on issues like housing, poll tax, and welfare rights.

Feminist Audio Books, 52–54 Featherstone Street, London EC1Y 8RT.
A tape subscription library for blind, partially sighted, and other women who have difficulty with the written word. Send sae for details.

Health Education Authority, Hamilton House, Mabledon Place, London WC1H 9TX. Tel. 071 383 3833.
The HEA is a special authority within the NHS with responsibility for providing advice and support about health education to the general public. They publish a very

wide range of health education resources, some specifically aimed at women – and many of their leaflets and booklets are free. Their catalogue includes a list of district health education units, which should stock HEA publications. HEA *What we publish* (1991) is available from the above address.

Health Rights Limited, Unit 110, Bon Marche Building, 444 Brixton Road, London SW9 8EJ. Tel. 071 274 4000, ext. 442.
Offer advice and information on health rights.

Help for Health Trust, High Croft Cottage, Romsey Road, Winchester SO22 5DH. Tel. 0962 849100.
Provides information on all aspects of health, with a database of thousands of support groups/self-help networks nationally. Subscription to the newsletter is £5 per annum and they sell information sheets on 65 different topics at a cost of 40p each. Send sae.

HMSO, Publications Centre, P.O. Box 276, London SW8 5DT.
HMSO stock all official government reports, parliamentary legislation, white papers, and so on. For example, they have new bills like the *Human Embryology and Fertilisation Bill*, which could be of interest to a group looking at abortion legislation.

Institute for Complementary Medicine, 21 Portland Place, London, W1N 3AF. Tel. 071 636 9543.
Provides information on complementary or alternative medicine, including details of local practitioners.

London Food Commission, 88 Old Street, London EC1V 9AR. Tel. 071 253 9513.
Stocks low cost leaflets and the like on food and health – send sae for publications list.

MIND (National Association for Mental Health), 22 Harley Street, London W1N 2ED. Tel. 071 637 0741.
Leaflets, information, details of local associations, and self-help groups concerned with all aspects of mental health, including women and mental health, and Black and minority ethnic mental health.

National Alliance of Women, 122 Whitechapel High Street, London E1 7PT. Tel. 071 247 7052.
Umbrella organisation acting as an advocate and support for all women's organisations nationally. Publishes regular mailings and offers networking, advice on fundraising, runs workshops, information exchange, and practical help. Membership costs £15–£20.

National Community Health Resource, 57 Chalton Street, London NW1 1HU. Tel. 071 383 3841.

Promotes community health initiatives, provides wide range of information, and publishes quarterly journal *Community Health Action*. NCHR also co-ordinates two national projects: Black Health Forum and Women's Health Network. NCHR organises regional and national training events, conferences and seminars. Membership costs £10–£16 for unfunded groups and includes subscriptions to the journal and bulletin. Write for publications list.

National Council for Voluntary Organisations, Regents Wharf, 8 All Saints Street, London N1 9RL.
Valuable source of information and publications on all aspects of voluntary organisations/services. Has a number of units working on special topics, for example, rural areas, local development, policy, community care, management, and so on. Write with sae for publications list.

National Federation of Women's Institutes, 104 New Kings Road, London SW6 4LY. Tel. 071 371 9300.
There are branches of the WI in small towns and villages throughout the country, often in rural areas where there are few other resources for women – it is worth contacting your local branch when planning or publicising events. The WI has a strong commitment to education and to women's health issues, a fact which many people are unaware of. The National Federation of Women's Institutes publishes a wide range of publications and a newsletter which costs £2.80 per year.

National Network of Local Information Services for Children, c/o Daycare Trust, Wesley House, 4 Wild Court, London WC2B 5AU. Tel. 071 405 5617.
This network is just emerging and aims to provide information and develop childcare provision at a local level, as well as providing a newsletter.

National Self-Help Support Centre, NCVO, 26 Bedford Square, London WC1B 3HU.
The National Self-Help Support Centre has published a number of guidelines which are useful for new groups and women who are not used to group working, including *Difficult members*, *Leadership in a self-help group* and *Coping with conflict*. Leaflets are free with a large (A4) sae.

National Union of Public Employees (NUPE), Civic House, 20 Grand Depot Road, Woolwich, London SE18 6SF. Tel. 071 854 2244.
NUPE publishes a looseleaf pack of leaflets on women's health called *Women's health matters*. They are clear and concise and a helpful basis for discussing unfamiliar topics with a new group.

NCHR Black Health Unit, 57 Chalton Street, London NW1 1HU. Tel. 071 383 3841. This is part of the National Community Health Resource.

Office of Health Economics, 12 Whitehall, London SW1A 2DY.
The OHE has published a useful summary of women's health issues called *Women's health today* (£1) and many other useful reasonably priced publications, for example, understanding the NHS, disability, and so on. Write for publications list.

Pre-school Playgroups Association, 61 Kings Cross Road, London WC1X 9LL.
Useful source of information on setting up a playgroup, some of which could be helpful to women who have to plan a crèche.

Trades Union Congress, Congress House, Great Russell Street, London WC1B 3LS. Tel. 071 636 4030.
The TUC can provide details of branches, activities and membership of all the unions affiliated to it. It also runs courses, publishes information leaflets on all aspects of health, welfare and safety at work, and has a library. Some trade unions now have women officers.

Wellbeing, The Volunteer Centre, 25–7 Elmbank Street, Glasgow G2 4PB. Tel. 041 226 3431.
Provides advice and information on health issues for both professionals and the general public, with extensive list of Scottish contacts.

Women's Aid Federation, P.O. Box 391, Bristol BS99 7WS. Tel. 0272 633494. (Helpline, Tel. 0272 633542.)
Provides information, leaflets (30p each or free), training packs, videos and books on domestic violence and related legal issues.

Women's Health (formerly WHRRIC), 52 Featherstone Street, London EC1Y 8RT. Tel. 071 251 6580.
Stocks a very wide selection of leaflets providing clear information on such topics as menopause, hormone replacement therapy, AIDS/HIV, and abnormal smears. Leaflets cost 30p–40p each, plus sae, and some are available in different Asian languages.

Women's Health Network, NCHR, 57 Chalton Street, London NW1 1HU. Tel. 071 383 3841.
National network providing information, support, and training for women health workers, that is any woman or group wanting to empower women to take control of their own health care. Also provides advice on funding, evaluation, administration and moving forward. WHN have a special commitment to rural women and black and minority ethnic women. Annual subscription to newsletter is £5 for unfunded groups and individuals, and £12 for funded groups. WHN also aims to support and develop regional networks. An invaluable source for new and established groups.

Women's Sports Foundation, c/o London Women's Centre, Wesley House, 4 Wild Court, London WC2B 5AU. Tel. 071 831 7863.
Dedicated to encouraging and promoting sporting activities for women – publishes leaflets, careers pack, and hires out exhibition and video on women and sport. Send sae for details.

Materials for training

Not everyone has access to flipcharts, paper, markers, post-its, and so on. Section 10 gives ideas where you might go for help with these. Here are some 'trainer's tips':

- Alternatives to flipchart pads
  - Paint shops and DIY superstores sell lining paper (for walls). It comes in large rolls, is much cheaper than buying flipcharts, and you can cut to the size you want.
  - You could approach your local newspaper and ask for end rolls of newsprint. These are the blank ends of the paper used for printing. You should get them free!
- Flipchart markers
  These are very easy to *lose* during a training session, especially if women are using them in small groups. You could put your name on a label on each one; know how many you had at the beginning, and at the end make sure everyone hands them in.
- Blu-tack
  The stuff for sticking paper to walls, and the like, can be carefully recycled by removing from flipcharts at end of session and using again and again.
- General stationery
  Many towns have *cheap* 'everyday' stationery shops, which are cheaper than going to an office supplies shop. You should be able to obtain more cheaply such things as small cards/glue/Blu-tack/post-it notes/paper, and so on.

Trainer's box of tricks

It can be very useful always to have with you on training sessions a box containing such things as:

- spare paper;
- flipchart markers;
- pens;
- envelopes of different sizes;
- Blu-tack;
- sellotape;
- Pritt Stick or roller glue;
- paper clips;
- stapler;
- post-it notes of different sizes and colours;
- small index cards;
- A5 size index cards – different colours;
- screwdriver;
- extension lead;
- ball of string;
- soft ball;
- folders;
- 'pinger' (i.e. one of those timers that you can set to ping after several minutes – useful for activities when you want people to change round after a certain time);
- small first aid kit;
- pain killers;
- sanitary towels and tampons;
- tissues/toilet roll;
- a few children's toys/paper/felt-tips/books, and so on (in case a child won't stay in the crèche and comes looking for mum!).

Trainers box of tricks

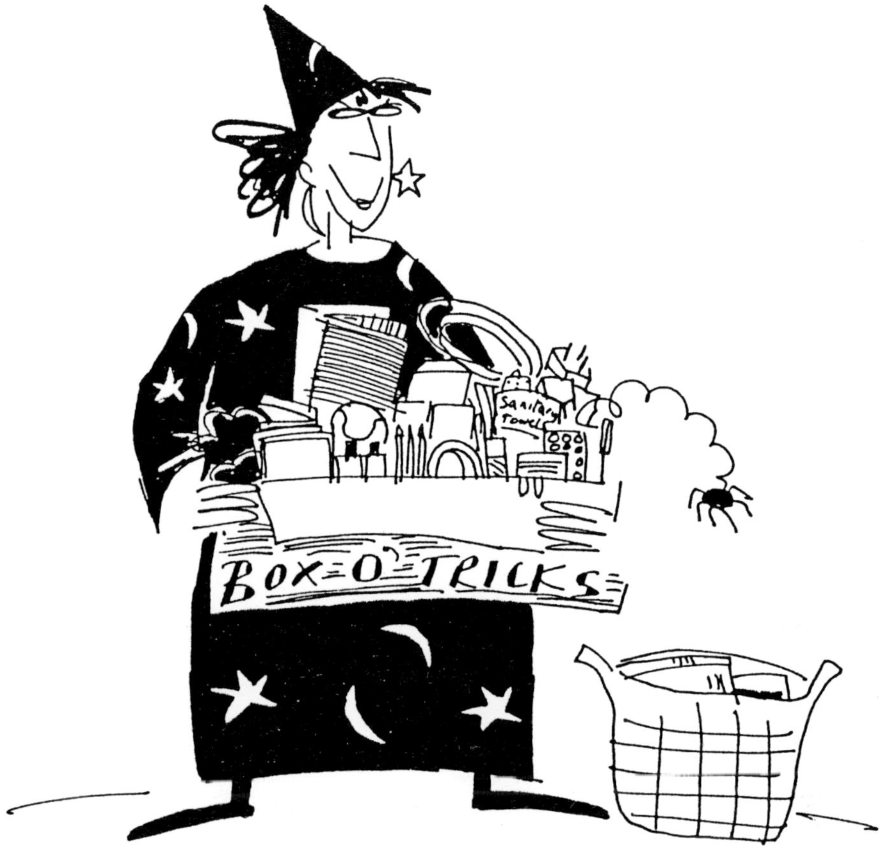

INDEX

Activities

Building on existing skills

Section 6
management and organisation in women's lives, 88

Section 8
how others see me, 178
validating and building on existing skills, 178
acknowledging existing skills, 183

Clarifying and strategising

Section 8
stepping stones, 209
SLOT, 210
moving forward – action wheel, 212
where next? 214

Closing

Section 8
something I'm looking forward to/going back to, 163
what I can do, 167
thunderstorm, 168
positive strokes I, 169
positive strokes II, 170

Differences and discrimination

Section 4
stereotyping between women, 45
similarities and differences, 47
differences between us, 48

Section 5
looking at sexism, 56
looking at racism, 60
how race can affect women's health, 63
heterosexism/homophobia, 66
images of lesbians, 68
looking at ageism, 72
looking at the health and health care of lesbians, 69
lifeline, 74
looking at disablism, 76

Evaluation

Section 7
why evaluate? 121
feelings about evaluation, 123
how to evaluate a women's health event, 127

Section 8

field of words, 156
evaluation round, 158
evaluation guided fantasy, 159
evaluation in small groups, 159
post-its, 162
something I'm taking away, 163
evaluation sheet 1, 164
evaluation sheet 2, 166

Expectations
Section 8
round, 142
index cards, 143
what I want from this event, 143

Games using small cards

Section 8
contraception game, 171
exploring dependencies, 173
symptoms of stress, 175
safer sex... HIV/AIDS, 176

Groupwork

Section 4
why work with groups? 43

Section 6
learning in groups, 84
role of tutor, 101

Section 8
why groupwork? 184
roles in groups, 186
goldfish bowl, 189
what helps a group work well, 190
role of tutor, 191
feelings about tutoring, 191
difficulties/roles in groups, 194
I can sabotage this group . . ., 195
case-studies of problems in groups, 196

Introductions

Section 8
names, 137
ballgame, 138
paired introductions, 138
fantasy introductions, 139
telling the truth, 141
what I want to be when I grow up, 141

Mood lighteners

Section 8
fruitbowl, 149
imaginary hat, 150
milling, 151
into a corner, 152
singing, 152
massage I, 153
massage II, 154
relaxation techniques, 155

Networking

Section 8
what is networking? I, 214
what is networking? II, 220

Organising sessions
Section 10
back to life, back to reality, 265
gaining support for training, 268

Planning sessions

Section 8
planning teaching sessions I, 201
planning teaching sessions II, 201
planning a course – who decides? 205
planning for problems – first meeting, 205
planning for problems – greatest fear, 208

Section 9
planning women's health events, 232
jigsaw frameworks, 235

Support

Section 8
my support group, 222
support please, 222

Training

Section 3
education and training, 20
what is training in women's health education?, 21
case-study on training, 23
different ways of training, 27
value of training, 29
good practice in training, 31

Section 10
back to life, back to reality, 265
gaining support for training, 268

Trust

Section 8
ground rules I, 145
ground rules II – brick wall, 146
things you never knew about me, 147
trust me, 148
snapshot, 148

Working with women and health

Section 4
why women only?, 38
why women and health?, 40
stereotyping between women, 45
similarities and differences, 47
differences between us, 48

Section 5
how race can affect women's health, 63
looking at the health and health care of lesbians, 69

Section 6
working with women, 91

INDEX

General

Activities

activities – different kinds of, 137
explanation of, 7
for training others *see* section 8, 177–225
process-based activities *see* section 8, 137–71
see Activities index

Ageism, 54

activity: looking at ageism, 72
activity: lifeline, 74
see Resources *in* section 5, 79

Case studies

case study on training, 23
developing women's health training, 276
difficult situations in groups, 197–200
role of the tutor, 102–3

Checklists

checklist of good practice, 107
final preparation, 99
training; checklist of good practice, 31–2
what helps a group work well, 190

Community health councils, 270, 274–5, 294

Crèche

crèche provision, 96
crèche workers, 275
example of a separate crèche form, 283
see childcare *in* section 11, 300

Co-working, 28

co-tutor, 17

Co-contracts, 273

example for evaluating each other, 288
example for organising events, 286
example for running event, 287

Directories, 296–7

Disability, 54

activity: looking at disablism, 76
see Resources *in* section 5, 80

Discrimination, 53

Differences
see **Women**

Evaluation

activity: feelings about evaluation, 123
activity: how to evaluate a women's health event, 127
activity: why evaluate, 121
evaluating yourself as a tutor, 131
evaluation by participants, 128
evaluation sheet, 323
judging success, 108
process of evaluation, 120
what is evaluation, 118
what to evaluate, 125
what to do with the evaluation, 132
when to evaluate, 127
who is evaluation for?, 125
who should evaluate, 126
see evaluation activities *in* section 8, 121–25, 127–8
see section 7, 115–34

Funding

costing and funding, 95, 264, 269, 275

Frameworks for training events

see section 9, 230–60
see **Groups, Organising events, Planning sessions**

Glossary, 16

Ground rules, 10

activity: ground rules I, 145
activity: ground rules II – brick wall, 146
definition of, 17

Groups

definitions of groupwork, 17
framework: groupwork I, 249
framework, groupwork II, 249
framework: two-day workshop on women's health and groupwork, 251
the group process (info. sheet), 112
ways of learning: groupwork and formal teaching methods (info. sheet), 33
see groupwork activities *in* Activities index, 312

Handbook

aims, 1
how developed, 1
organisation of, 5
routes through, 12
using, 4

Heterosexism, 54

activity: images of lesbians, 68
activity: looking at heterosexism and homophobia, 66
activity: looking at the health and health care of lesbians, 69

Health promotion units, 270, 274–5, 276, 294

Learning

activity: learning in groups, 84
cycle of competence, 110
from experience, 84
from others, 93
how people learn (info. sheet), 111
ways of learning: groupwork and formal teaching methods (info. sheet), 33
see section 6, 82–114

Lesbians

activity: images of lesbians, 68
activity: looking at the health and health care of lesbians, 69

Micro-teaching, 17, 28

Networking, 28

activity: what is networking I, 214
activity: what is networking II, 220

Opportunities for training

developing women's health training, 276
see section 10, 261–292

Organisations

collaborating with other organisations, 270
meeting your needs relating to training events, 274–5
training within an organisation, 274
see organisations *in* section 11, 302

Organising events

activity: management and organisation, 88
frameworks for women's health training, 230–60
organising events, 93
running events, 100

Planning sessions

course over a number of weeks, 235
one-day event, 232
residential event, 234
two-day event, 234
two-hour session, 232
see section 9, 230–60
see planning sessions activities *in* Activities index, 313

Problems

activity: back to life, back to reality, 265
activity: case studies of problems in groups, 196
activity: difficulties and roles in groups, 194
activity: gaining support for training, 268
activity: I could sabotage this group by . . . , 195
activity: planning for problems: my greatest fear, 208
activity: planning for problems: the first meeting, 205
activity: role of the tutor (case studies), 101
organising events, 93
problem solving: when things go wrong, 257
setting the scene – opportunities for training, 264

Publicity

calendar of religious/cultural festivals, 289
example of a registration form, 282
example of letter to be sent out upon receipt of registration form, 284
points to remember when publicising an event, 277
samples of publicity, 280–1

Race

see Resources *in* section 5, 78

Racism, 53

activity: how race can affect women's health, 63
activity: looking at racism, 60

Religious/cultural festivals

calendar of religious/cultural festivals, 289–90

Registration

see **Publicity**

Resources

see section 11, 293–309
books and packs, 298
bookshops (mail order books), 302
directories, 296
films and videos, 301
local resources, 293
materials for training, 307
organisations, 302
trainers box of tricks, 308
see Resources at end of each section

Sessions

follow-up sessions, 252
frameworks for women's health training *see* section 9, 230–60
running sessions *see* section 8, 135–229
structuring sessions, 98

Sexism, 53

activity: looking at sexism, 56

Sexuality

see Resources in section 5, 80
see **Heterosexism, Lesbians**

Support

activity: my support group, 222
activity: support please!, 222

Teaching/learning methods, 13

adapting a teaching method for different topics, 171
ways of learning: groupwork and formal teaching methods (info. sheet), 33
see section 8 for examples of different teaching methods, 135–229

Training

activity: gaining support for training, 268
developing women's health training (case studies), 276
framework: training issues, 250
introducing training, 9
materials for training, 307
opportunities for training *see* section 10, 261–92
trainers box of tricks, 308
training others *see* section 8, 177–225
see section 3, 18–35
see section 11, 293–309
see training activities *in* Activities index, 313

Tutor

activity: role of the tutor, 191
activity: the role of the tutor, 101
definition of, 17
role of tutor/facilitator, 10

Well-women centres, 270, 274–5, 276, 294

Worksheets

acknowledging and building on existing skills, 183
action wheel, 213
action worksheet A, 215
action worksheet B, 216
action worksheet C, 217
back to life, back to reality, 267
cartoon: feelings about tutoring/leading groups, 193
case studies of problems in groups, 197–200
case-study on training, 23
case-studies of the role of the tutor, 102–3
evaluation: field of words, 157
evaluation in small groups, 161
grid of skills and talents, 180–2
how race can affect women's health, 64
learning in groups, 85
looking at ageism, 73

looking at the health and health care of lesbians, 70
looking at heterosexism and homophobia, 67
management and organisation, 90
my support group, 223
planning a course: who decides, 206
planning teaching sessions, 202–4
racist remarks, 61–2
roles in groups, 187–8
role of the tutor, 192
sexist remarks, 57–9
SLOT exercise, 211
stereotyping between women, 46
strengths and weaknesses, 179
support please, 224
the first meeting, 207
using the *Women and Health* pack I, 248
using the *Women and Health* pack II, 245
what do you need to think about when planning, 233
what is networking?, 219
what I want from this event, 144
why women and health?, 41
why women only?, 39
working with women, 92

Women

activity: working with women, 91
differences between
see section 4, 45–9
see section 5, 52–81
framework: using the *Women and Health* pack I, 242
framework: using the *Women and Health* pack II, 243
framework: women's health and groupwork I, 246
framework: women's health and groupwork II, 247
framework: women's health tutor training course, 255
framework: two-day workshop on women's health and groupwork, 251
working with, section 4, 36–51
see section 11, 293–309
see working with women and health activities, *in* Activities index, 314

Evaluation sheet

Your comments

We are interested in finding out *who* is using this handbook, *in what way* it is being used, and *how it could be improved* in any future edition. Your comments would therefore be very much appreciated.

Please send a copy of the completed form on the following pages back to:

The Women's Health Officer
Health Education Authority,
Hamilton House,
Mabledon Place,
London WC1H 9TX.

Evaluation Sheet:

Women together: A health education training handbook for ourselves and others.

Your name, address, organisation (optional)

1. Where did you first hear about this handbook?

2. Have you used this handbook as a training resource *for yourself*? Yes/no
   please explain

3. Have you used this handbook as a resource for training *others*? Yes/no
   please explain

4. • *With whom* have you used the handbook?
   (e.g. adult education students, midwives, young women, health promotion officers).

   • *What* was the event you were running?
   (e.g. women's health course, one-off session, two-day workshop, training session on groupwork skills).

5. Have you found the handbook:
   • Easy to use in finding what you wanted? Yes/no
   please explain.

   • Easy to use in terms of layout? Yes/no
   please explain.

- Easy to understand? Yes/no
  please explain.

- Appropriate for the particular group you have used the handbook with? Yes/no
  please explain.

6. Are there any *sections* that you have found particularly useful (e.g. Working with women, learning from experience)?

7. Are there any *activities* and/or *worksheets* that you have found particularly useful (e.g. SLOT activity, 'Jigsaw game')?

8. Are the *resources* adequate?
   Suggestions for further resources to be included:

9. Is there anything else you would like the handbook to cover?

10. Any other comments you would like to make?

Thank you for filling this in